CRITICAL ISSUES IN SCHOOL-BASED MENTAL HEALTH

School-based mental health professionals intervene daily to address a variety of student mental health concerns. From challenges that arise in the educational context to those carried over from home, from managing daily care to handling emergent traumatic events, they must be prepared for an extremely varied work life. While some of the most common issues recur with such frequency that they may seem straightforward to address, others crop up with changing student populations.

Each chapter in this volume addresses a different key topic, giving current and future professionals an overview of the most recent scholarship on the topic, and then outlining evidence-based interventions. With chapters on learning disabilities, substance abuse, bullying, internalizing and externalizing behaviors, trauma, LGBTQ youth, and more, this book prepares school-based mental health professionals to face some of the most difficult, common, and politicized issues affecting students today.

Melissa K. Holt is Assistant Professor in Counseling Psychology in the School of Education at Boston University, USA.

Amie E. Grills is Associate Professor in Counseling Psychology in the School of Education at Boston University, USA.

CRITICAL ISSUES IN SCHOOL-BASED MENTAL HEALTH

Evidence-based Research, Practice, and Interventions

Edited by Melissa K. Holt and Amie E. Grills

Routledge
Taylor & Francis Group
NEW YORK AND LONDON

First published 2016
by Routledge
711 Third Avenue, New York, NY 10017

and by Routledge
2 Park Square, Milton Park, Abingdon, Oxon OX14 4RN

Routledge is an imprint of the Taylor & Francis Group, an informa business

Library of Congress Cataloging-in-Publication Data
Names: Holt, Melissa K., editor. | Grills, Amie E., editor.
Title: Critical issues in school-based mental health : evidence-based research, practice, and interventions / edited by Melissa K. Holt and Amie E. Grills.
Description: New York, NY : Routledge, 2016. | Includes bibliographical references and index.
Identifiers: LCCN 2015024658 |
Subjects: LCSH: School children—Mental health services—United States. | School health services—United States. | School psychology—United States.
Classification: LCC LB3430 .C75 2016 | DDC 371.7/13—dc23
LC record available at http://lccn.loc.gov/2015024658

ISBN: 978-1-138-02500-4 (hbk)
ISBN: 978-1-138-02501-1 (pbk)
ISBN: 978-1-315-77542-5 (ebk)

Typeset in Bembo
by Apex CoVantage, LLC

CONTENTS

ACKNOWLEDGMENTS

Thank you to our editor, Rebecca Novack, for her commitment to this project, and to Trevor Gori and Daniel Schwartz for their guidance through the publication process. We also would like to acknowledge and thank all of the authors who contributed their time and care into preparing the exceptional chapters included in this book. Finally, we would like to express our gratitude to the many individuals working in schools every day to improve the quality of children's lives.

–MH & AG

To my parents, John and Barbara, who were proud of even the first books I created with construction paper and crayons—thank you for instilling the value of education and hard work. To my husband, Lowell, this book would not have been possible without your steadfast support and encouragement—thank you for the lightness you bring into my life. Finally, this book is dedicated to my children: Nicholas (11), for our nightly conversations, which mean the world to me; Katherine (8), for your beautiful (and sparkly) notes of encouragement; and Emmeline (7 months), for your infectious smile and giggle.

–MH

For your support and ability to make me smile after the longest of days, I dedicate this book to my partner, Nate, and to my girls—

Frankie (age 6), you told me that, if I were famous, it would be for working hard to help kids.

Lucy (age 2), you told me that I have hair like Rapunzel (and then pulled some out).

While I will never be famous or a princess, I am far more fortunate to have the endless joy and love you bring to my life.

–AG

1

INTRODUCTION: ADDRESSING YOUTH MENTAL HEALTH IN SCHOOLS

Melissa K. Holt and Amie E. Grills

Approximately one in five youth experience a mental health disorder (President's New Freedom Commission on Mental Health, 2003). In turn, mental health disorders are associated with a host of problems in other domains (e.g., academic and social adjustment difficulties), the combination of which can compromise optimal development (Suldo, Gormley, DuPaul, & Anderson-Butcher, 2014; van Lier et al., 2012). As detailed throughout this book, multiple evidence-based treatment and prevention approaches have been identified that can buffer deleterious effects of mental health disorders and their comorbid challenges. However, despite recent increases in service use for mental disorders among youth (Perou et al., 2013), the majority of youth do not receive mental health services (Merikangas et al., 2011). Moreover, there are significant disparities in mental health access and quality; racial/ethnic minority and low socioeconomic status (SES) youth, as well as uninsured youth, receive treatment at particularly low rates (Merikangas et al., 2011). Given the current landscape of youth mental health issues in the United States, schools are increasingly being called upon to play integral roles in the identification of mental health concerns and provision of mental health services. In this Introduction, we briefly consider schools' role in light of a social-ecological framework and provide an overview of topics covered in subsequent chapters.

The Role of Schools in Addressing Mental Health

The social-ecological perspective highlights that youth behaviors and functioning are shaped by both individual characteristics and a range of nested contextual systems, such as schools, families, and neighborhoods (Bronfenbrenner, 1977). Each of these systems interacts with the others and, singularly and in combination, influences youth development. The framework, when applied to youth mental health, suggests that while individual characteristics (e.g., genetic factors) might predispose a youth to experience mental health concerns, influences from other systems can serve to promote psychological health or, conversely, contribute to the maintenance of psychological distress.

Given that youth spend a significant amount of time in school, schools represent a key context for the identification of mental health issues, intervention, and prevention. Indeed, in the President's New Freedom Commission on Mental Health, the enhancement of school-based mental health services was identified as a crucial mechanism for improving early screening and connection to appropriate services (President's New Freedom Commission on Mental Health, 2003). President Obama further highlighted the role teachers specifically can play in helping to identify youth who might be experiencing mental health problems and proposed funding to improve teacher training in this area (The White House, 2013). For instance, teachers may be able to serve as student advocates if they receive appropriate education and training around how to recognize warning signs of mental illness and distress in their students. In this manner, teachers might serve as an important referral source for further student evaluation by trained professionals who could then delineate appropriate services (Jensen et al., 2011). Importantly, schools are particularly well positioned to reach traditionally underserved populations (Owens, Murphy, Richerson, Girio, & Himawan, 2008), offering a point of contact for youth who might otherwise not have their mental health concerns addressed.

Efforts to respond to mental health issues in school settings have shown significant promise, as the authors of each chapter in this book delineate. Research suggests that even the availability of school-based mental health programs can make a difference; when these are available, not only are youth more likely to report seeing a counselor within the past year, but there is also evidence that there are not racial/ethnic disparities in accessing these services (Slade, 2002). Following the social-ecological framework, scholars have argued for an expansion of school-based mental health programs, such that schools and community programs and agencies work in collaboration with families to respond to youth mental health concerns (Weist & Evans, 2005). Similarly, in the ecological model set forth by Doll and colleagues (Doll, Spies, & Champion, 2012), they highlight that in contrast to the traditional approach to school mental health services that draws from the medical model, the ecological approach allows for a better integration of systems, from classrooms to schools to families. This, in turn, is responsive to the fact that multiple levels of the social ecology influence mental health concerns.

Overview of Chapters

Taken together, chapters in this book provide a comprehensive source of information on key issues school-based mental health professionals will encounter and need to address. Within each chapter, authors attend to relevant social-ecological dimensions, with particular attention to developmental considerations, gender, and race/ethnicity. Further, authors provide information about evidence-based assessment, treatment, intervention, and prevention approaches, and highlight relevant resources for professionals working in schools.

The first six chapters cover primary disorders experienced by school-aged youth (Chapter 2—Externalizing Behaviors; Chapter 3—Internalizing Behaviors; Chapter 4—Learning Disabilities; Chapter 5—Autism Spectrum Disorder; Chapter 6—Substance Use; Chapter 7—Eating Disorders and Obesity). Subsequently, five chapters discuss issues that are particularly relevant during youth development and provide contemporary information important for school professionals. Moreover, these topics reflect ones which to date have received limited attention in books focused on school mental health and services (Chapter 8—Health Issues; Chapter 9—Sexuality; Chapter 10—LBGTQ Youth; Chapter 12—Bullying; Chapter 13—Dating and Sexual Violence). Given the importance of the social-ecological system, other chapters focus on family and community domains as well as their intersection with schools (Chapter 11—Family Adjustment Issues; Chapter 14—Effects of Childhood Trauma; Chapter 15—Family Engagement). Finally, a Universal Prevention Model (Chapter 16) is presented to bring together assessment and prevention themes from previous chapters and to highlight a model for schools to effectively address mental health concerns among students.

Given the number of youth affected by mental health concerns, and the unmet needs of many of these individuals, schools represent one key context in which mental health concerns can be assessed and addressed, and in which optimal development can be promoted.

References

Bronfenbrenner, U. (1977). Toward an experimental ecology of human development. *American Psychologist, 32*, 513–531.

Doll, B., Spies, R., & Champion, A. (2012). Contributions of ecological school mental health services to students' academic success. *Journal of Educational & Psychological Consultation, 22*(1–2), 44–61. doi: 10.1080/10474412.2011.649642

Jensen, P.S., Goldman, E., Offord, D., Costello, E.J., Friedman, R., Huff, B., . . . Roberts, R. (2011). Overlooked and underserved: 'Action signs' for identifying children with unmet mental health needs. *Pediatrics, 128*(5), 970–979. doi: 10.1542/peds.2009–0367

Merikangas, K.R., He, J.-P., Burstein, M., Swendsen, J., Avenevoli, S., Case, B., . . . Olfson, M. (2011). Service utilization for lifetime mental disorders in U.S. Adolescents: Results of the National Comorbidity Survey-Adolescent Supplement (NCSA). *Journal of the American Academy of Child & Adolescent Psychiatry, 50*(1), 32–45. doi: 10.1016/j.jaac.2010.10.006

Owens, J. S., Murphy, C. E., Richerson, L., Girio, E. L., & Himawan, L. K. (2008). Science to practice in underserved communities: The effectiveness of school mental health programming. *Journal of Clinical Child and Adolescent Psychology, 37*(2), 434–447. doi: 10.1080/15374410801955912

Perou, R., Bitsko, R.H., Blumberg, S.J., Pastor, P., Ghandour, R. M., Gfroerer, J.C., . . . Huang, L.N. (2013). Mental health surveillance among children—United States, 2005–2011. *Morbidity and Mortality Weekly Report, 62*(2), 1–35.

President's New Freedom Commission on Mental Health. (2003). *Achieving the promise: Transforming mental health care in America. Final report*. Rockville, MD: Department of Health and Human Services.

Slade, E.P. (2002). Effects of school-based mental health programs on mental health service use by adolescents at school and in the community. *Mental Health Services Research, 4*(3), 151–166. doi: 10.1023/A:1019711113312

Suldo, S.M., Gormley, M.J., DuPaul, G.J., & Anderson-Butcher, D. (2014). The impact of school mental health on student and school-level academic outcomes: Current status of the research and future directions. *School Mental Health, 6*(2), 84–98. doi: 10.1007/s12310–013–9116–2

The White House. (2013). Presidential proclamation: National Mental Health Awareness Month, 2013. Retrieved from http://www.whitehouse.gov/the-press-office/2013/04/30/presidential-proclamation-national-mental-health-awareness-month-2013

van Lier, P.A.C., Vitaro, F., Barker, E.D., Brendgen, M., Tremblay, R.E., & Boivin, M. (2012). Peer victimization, poor academic achievement, and the link between childhood externalizing and internalizing problems. *Child Development, 83*(5), 1775–1788. doi: 10.1111/j.1467–8624.2012.01802.x

Weist, M.D., & Evans, S.W. (2005). Expanded school mental health: Challenges and opportunities in an emerging field. *Journal of Youth and Adolescence, 34*(1), 3–6. doi: 10.1007/s10964–005–1330–2

2

EXTERNALIZING BEHAVIORS

Nicole P. Powell, John E. Lochman, Caroline L. Boxmeyer, and Meghann K. Sallee

Externalizing behaviors include aggression and conduct problems. Aggression is generally defined as a behavioral act that results in harming or hurting others. Because aggressive behavior and its treatment vary greatly according to the intentions and conditions surrounding the aggression, it is typically categorized according to different types. Aggression can be physical or verbal; relational, proactive, or reactive; and overt or covert. The literature often differentiates between proactive and reactive aggression because such a framework allows for the explanation and description of aggression (Dodge, Lochman, Harnish, Bates, & Pettit, 1997). Children engaging in proactive aggression typically use aggression to meet a goal. When the aggressive behavior yields the desired reward, the child is more likely to engage in proactive aggression the next time s/he intends to meet a goal. Conversely, reactively aggressive children do not seek to meet goals through their aggression. Instead, these children react quickly and impulsively to perceived or actual threats and can become intensely irritated.

From a psychodiagnostic perspective, Disruptive Behavior Disorders are clinical manifestations of externalizing behavior problems. Oppositional Defiant Disorder (ODD) involves angry and irritable mood, argumentative and defiant behavior, and vindictiveness. Prevalence rates for ODD range from 1% to 11% (American Psychiatric Association, 2013), with age of onset starting at around

---

Authors' Note: The preparation of this chapter was supported by grants from the National Institute of Child Health and Human Development (R01HD079273), the National Institute on Drug Abuse (R34 DA034295), and the U.S. Department of Education (R305A140070). Correspondence concerning this chapter should be directed to Dr. Nicole Powell, Center for the Prevention of Youth Behavior Problems, The University of Alabama, Tuscaloosa, AL 35487–0348.

four years of age and steadily increasing through late adolescence (Nock, Kazdin, Hiripi, & Kessler, 2007). In childhood, the disorder appears to be somewhat more common in boys (1.4:1), though prevalence rates do not vary by gender in adolescents or adults (American Psychiatric Association, 2013). Few changes to the Diagnostic and Statistical Manual of Mental Disorders, 4th Edition, Text Revision (DSM-IV TR) diagnostic criteria for ODD were made with the publication of *Diagnostic and Statistical Manual of Mental Disorders* (DSM-5). While the DSM-IV TR symptom list was retained, DSM-5 adds a specification that symptomatic behaviors must occur outside of sibling relationships, provides guidance for distinguishing normative vs. symptomatic behaviors for children younger than 5 years and those 5 years or older, and includes severity specifiers related to the number of settings in which problematic behaviors occur.

Conduct Disorder (CD) is prevalent in 4% of youth, and is more prevalent in boys than girls, at a rate of about 3 to 1 (prevalence of 6–16% for boys and 2–9% for girls). DSM-5 criteria for CD include four sets of symptoms involving aggression towards others, destruction of property, covert behaviors such as lying and stealing, and serious violations of rules (running away from home, truant from school; American Psychiatric Association, 2013). These symptoms are unchanged from DSM-IV TR. Also consistent with DSM-IV TR, DSM-5 criteria provide for three levels of severity of CD, with the most severe involving primarily aggressive symptoms.

In both DSM-IV TR and DSM-5, CD can be specified by age of onset. Childhood-onset CD begins prior to age 10 years, and adolescent-onset CD is asymptomatic until after age 10. The latter form of CD is expected to remit by adulthood for most adolescents. In contrast, youth with childhood-onset CD are typically more aggressive and have increased and persistent rates of criminal behavior and substance-related disorders throughout adolescence and adulthood. Most children who meet criteria for childhood-onset CD also meet criteria for ODD and have notable difficulties with peers. DSM-5 also includes specifiers focusing on limited prosocial emotions, lack of remorse or guilt, callousness and lack of empathy for others' feelings, lack of concern for poor performance in important activities, and shallow or deficient affect.

CD is associated with a wide range of negative outcomes in adolescence, including truancy, substance use, early teenage pregnancy, and delinquency (American Psychiatric Association, 2013). Youth with CD are at risk for later mood disorders, anxiety disorders, posttraumatic stress disorder, impulse control disorders, and psychotic disorders, as well as substance-related disorders as adults (American Psychiatric Association, 2013).

Children who are at risk for disruptive behavior problems can be identified at early ages in school settings (Essex et al., 2009). Disruptive behavior often co-occurs with poor academic functioning and lower levels of school connectedness (Bradshaw, Buckley, & Ialongo, 2008). Poor grades in middle school are among the strongest predictors of students' subsequent dropout from school, which in turn affects students' likelihood for adequate occupational and life adjustment (Bowers, 2010). Given schools' focus on academic instruction and the importance of academic skills to children's development (Masten, Desjardins, McCormick, Kuo, & Long, 2010), it is crucial to understand how prevention and intervention programs for disruptive behavior impact children's academic functioning. Although aggressive children have declining academic grades from grades 3 through 8, cognitive-behavioral interventions have reduced these children's dramatic decline in language arts grades by 60% (Lochman, Boxmeyer, & Powell, 2012).

Children with emotional and behavioral problems and other disabilities are eligible for special education services in their schools. During the 2003–2004 school year, over 484,000 students received special education and related services under the emotional disturbance classification, representing approximately 1% of students (U.S. Department of Education, 2007). Children with emotional and behavioral problems typically begin having trouble with their behavior during grade school and have increased conflict with family and peers as they develop (Smith, Lochman, & Daunic, 2005). On average, youth with emotional disturbances have considerably lower academic achievement scores in comparison to their peers who do not receive special education services (Wagner, Newman, Cameto, & Levine, 2006).

Etiological Factors

As described in the contextual social-cognitive framework (Matthys & Lochman, 2010), children can experience a "stacking" of risk factors as they develop, increasing the probability that they will eventual display serious antisocial behavior. These risk factors can be conceptualized as falling within several categories.

Biological and temperament factors. Some prenatal factors, such as maternal exposure to alcohol, methadone, cocaine, and cigarette smoke as well as severe nutritional deficiencies (Wakschlag, Pickett, Kasza, & Loeber, 2006), have been found to have direct effects on children's neurocognitive status and their subsequent aggression. Risk factors such as birth complications, genes, abnormal serotonin levels, and temperament can contribute to children's conduct problems, but only when environmental factors such as harsh parenting, interparental violence, or low socioeconomic status are present (Foley et al., 2004).

Community and neighborhood contextual factors. High neighborhood crime rates, low social cohesion, and neighborhood disadvantage have been found to predict disruptive behavior in children, especially proactive aggression (Fite, Wynn, Lochman, & Wells, 2009). Children's conduct problems can be exacerbated at school due to frustration with academic demands and negative peer influences. Classrooms characterized by disapproving teachers and disengaged students undermine the learning environment and can elicit children's disruptive behavior (Thomas, Bierman, Thompson, & Conduct Problems Prevention Research Group, 2008). The density of aggressive children in a classroom can increase the amount of aggression emitted by individual students (Barth, Dunlap, Dane, Lochman, & Wells, 2004).

Family contextual factors. Children's aggression has been linked to family factors such as parent criminality; substance use and depression; poverty; marital conflict; stressful life events; single and teenage parenthood; and ambivalent, controlling parent-child attachment (Lochman et al., 2012). These family risks can influence child behavior through their effect on parenting processes, as when high levels of maternal depression predict parents' use of inconsistent discipline, which in turn predicts children's aggressive behavior (Barry, Dunlap, Lochman, & Wells, 2009). Parenting processes linked to children's aggression (e.g., Reid, Patterson, & Snyder, 2002) include harsh, inconsistent discipline; unclear directions and commands; lack of warmth and involvement; and lack of parental supervision and monitoring.

Peer contextual factors. Aggressive children who are also socially rejected exhibit more severe antisocial behavior than children who are aggressive only or rejected only (Lochman & Wayland, 1994). As adolescents, youth with conduct problems tend to associate with deviant peers, even if they have been previously rejected by peers, increasing the probability that the seriousness of their antisocial behavior will escalate (e.g., Dishion, Andrews, & Crosby, 1995).

Social cognition. Based on children's temperament and biological dispositions, and on contextual experiences from their family, peers, and community, they begin to form stable patterns of processing social information and of regulating their emotions. The contextual social-cognitive model (Lochman & Wells, 2002a) stresses the reciprocal interactive relationships between children's cognitions about events and their physiological arousal (Williams, Lochman, Phillips, & Barry, 2003). Aggressive children can have cognitive distortions at the appraisal phases of social-cognitive processing because of difficulties in encoding incoming social information, partially due to neurocognitive difficulties in their executive functions (Ellis, Weiss, & Lochman, 2009), and in accurately interpreting social events and others' intentions. Aggressive children have been found to recall fewer relevant cues about events (Lochman & Dodge, 1994), and to misperceive the levels of aggression that they and peers emit in dyadic interactions (Lochman & Dodge, 1998). Reactively aggressive children have a hostile attributional bias, as they excessively infer that others are acting toward them in a hostile manner (Dodge et al., 1997; Orobio de Castro, Veerman, Koops, Bosch, & Monshouwer, 2002).

Aggressive children also can have cognitive deficiencies as they try to problem-solve. Their dominance and revenge-oriented social goals (Lochman, Wayland, & White, 1993) guide the maladaptive action-oriented and nonverbal solutions they generate for perceived problems (Lochman & Dodge, 1994). Aggressive children expect that aggression will lead to positive outcomes for them (Lochman & Dodge, 1994). Deficient beliefs at this stage of information processing are especially characteristic for children with proactive aggressive behavior patterns (Dodge et al., 1997) and callous-unemotional traits (Pardini, Lochman, & Frick, 2003).

Best Practices for Assessment and Identification

The collection of data from multiple informants, and from multiple instruments, is a hallmark of a comprehensive assessment and is necessary to examine the many aspects of disruptive behavior disorder diagnoses in children and adolescents, how problems are manifested in different settings, and associated features (e.g., problems with peers, declining school performance; Kazdin, 2005). A broad approach to assessment is also important in evaluating children and adolescents because youth often exhibit symptoms of multiple disorders or meet criteria for two or more conditions. ADHD, mood disorders, and substance use problems are some of the more frequently co-occurring issues with externalizing behaviors (Nock et al., 2007).

Collecting data from multiple informants can be complicated by discrepancies among reporters. Divergent reports can be a function of the setting—for example, when aggression is more frequently and severely expressed at home than at school (e.g., De Los Reyes, Henry, Tolan, & Wakschlag, 2009). In the school setting, methods such as functional analysis and/or observations may be useful for clarifying discrepant information.

Goals for assessment can include, but are not limited to, screening, evaluation of a targeted area of functioning, diagnostic clarification, and appraisal of a youth's progress in treatment or general developmental progress (Sattler, 2001). Screening and targeted evaluations tend to be brief and narrowly focused; results of such assessments are necessarily provisional and limited in scope. Diagnostic assessment reflects a comprehensive approach, incorporating evaluation of strengths and weaknesses across multiple areas of functioning. Ongoing assessment of treatment progress provides important feedback to clinicians that can improve the quality and efficiency of interventions.

Barry, Golmaryami, Rivera-Hudson, and Frick (2013) provide a useful review of assessment principles for youth conduct problems. First, assessment tools must be able to evaluate for a range of externalizing symptoms in terms of both type and severity. Second, assessments must screen for co-occurring symptoms and provide information about their relation to the child's conduct problems. Third, assessments must evaluate for risk and protective factors that may influence symptom presentation as well as the course of treatment. Fourth, to improve treatment specificity, assessments must provide information that will help to distinguish among subtypes of CD. A comprehensive assessment for conduct problems will include a structured interview such as the Diagnostic Interview Schedule for Children (DISC; Shaffer, Fisher, Lucas, Dulcan, & Schwab-Stone, 2000), broad-band (e.g., Behavior Assessment System for Children, 2nd Edition; Reynolds & Kamphaus, 2004) and narrow-band (e.g., Antisocial Process Screening

Device; Frick & Hare, 2001) rating scales, behavioral observation techniques, and performance-based measures to provide the specific information about a given child needed for accurate diagnosis and effective treatment planning (see Barry et al., 2013 for additional recommended assessment measures and methods). Further, these instruments should be administered and interpreted with attention to cultural factors that affect symptom presentation.

Evidence-based Intervention and Prevention

There are a number of effective intervention options that can be implemented within the school context for children who display externalizing problem behaviors. Three well-supported programs designed for delivery in the school setting include LifeSkills Training, Incredible Years, and Coping Power.

LifeSkills Training. The LifeSkills Training Program is a universal program designed to prevent adolescent substance abuse (Botvin & Kantor, 2000). The program consists of 15 sessions, intended for implementation during the first year of middle school. Booster sessions are then provided during the following two school years. The program uses cognitive-behavioral techniques to teach students about personal self-management, social skills, and drug resistance skills. Results from a series of randomized controlled efficacy trials and two effectiveness studies indicate the program is highly effective in reducing alcohol, tobacco, marijuana, and polydrug use. Evaluation results support the long-term effectiveness of the program as well as its generalizability to diverse geographic, socioeconomic, and racial/ethnic groups (Botvin & Griffin, 2004). Further, an expanded version of the program has been shown to have preventive effects on physical aggression, verbal aggression, and delinquency (Botvin & Griffin, 2004).

Incredible Years. Incredible Years (IY) is a series of programs targeting children ages 2 to 10 years that is designed to reduce childhood behavior problems and to increase social competence at home and at school (Webster-Stratton & Reid, 2003).

Incredible Years Parent program. The Incredible Years Parent program consists of 13 two-hour group parent sessions. Topics of sessions include positive parent-child interaction, effective discipline techniques, and teaching children problem-solving skills. The parent program has been shown to decrease negative parenting behaviors and increase overall positive interactions observed between parent and child (Webster-Stratton, Reid, & Hammond, 2004).

Incredible Years Child program. The Incredible Years Child program consists of 22 two-hour group sessions. The goal is to learn about problem solving and social skills. Research supports the child program being superior to waitlist control groups at reducing disruptive behavior. Significant improvements have been shown in problem solving and conflict management behaviors, reductions in problem behaviors at home, reductions in conduct problems and increased prosocial behavior with peers, and reductions in amount of aggression exhibited at school (Webster-Stratton & Hammond, 1997; Webster-Stratton et al., 2004, Webster-Stratton, Reid, & Hammond, 2001). An evaluation conducted within the elementary school setting with kindergarten through first grade students indicated positive effects on teacher-reported externalizing problems (Reid, Webster-Stratton, & Hammond, 2007). The inclusion of a parenting component resulted in additional benefits for children's emotion regulation and on mothers' use of positive parenting (Reid et al., 2007).

Incredible Years Teacher program. The Incredible Years Teacher program is intended to help increase positive teacher-child relationships. Teachers are taught strategies to help children learn anger management strategies and problem solving skills and increase children's appropriate social behaviors and their prosocial communication (Webster-Stratton & Reid, 2007). The teacher program has been shown to improve behavior management and decrease the report of problem behavior within the classroom (Webster-Stratton et al., 2004).

Coping Power. The Coping Power program is a school-based preventative intervention for children considered at-risk because of their aggressive behavior. The program targets children in 4th to 6th grade, but can be adapted for early adolescents (7th and 8th grade). Coping Power includes a 34-session child component and coordinated 16-session parent component, both designed for implementation over a 16- to 18-month period. The main areas of focus for the child component include goal setting, organization and study skills, emotion awareness, anger management, perspective taking, social problem-solving, and resisting peer pressure. Main content areas for the parent sessions include positive parenting skills, family cohesion and communication, family problem-solving, involvement in children's academic programs, and behavior management. The child and parent components are both based on the contextual social-cognitive model of risk for youth aggression (Lochman & Wells, 2002a).

Coping Power: Evidence base. An efficacy study of the Coping Power program randomly assigned 183 aggressive boys in the 4th and 5th grades to one of three conditions: (1) the Coping Power Child component (delivered at school), (2) Combined Coping Power Child and Parent Training components, and (3) an untreated cell. At the one-year follow-up, in comparison to the untreated condition, results indicated the combined intervention cell produced reductions in children's self-reported delinquent behavior, and in parent-reported alcohol and marijuana use by the child. Teacher-reported behavioral improvements in school seemed to be primarily influenced by the child component (Lochman & Wells, 2004).

Results from several effectiveness studies support intervention effects on aggressive behavior and problem solving skills among deaf children in a residential setting (Lochman et al., 2001); overt aggression with ODD or CD in Dutch outpatient clinics in comparison to care-as-usual children (van de Wiel et al., 2007); and lower rates of substance use, improvements in social competence with peers, and greater increases in problem solving and anger coping skills for children who received Coping Power plus classroom intervention compared to children who received classroom intervention alone (Lochman & Wells, 2002b). A one-year follow-up of the latter study found Coping Power adolescents to have lower rates of self-reported substance use and delinquency, and lower levels of teacher-rated aggressive social behavior at school when compared to the control adolescents (Lochman & Wells, 2003). A longer-term three-year follow-up provided support for reduction in externalizing behavior long after intervention ended (Lochman, Wells, Qu, & Chen, 2013). In a dissemination study, Coping Power was found to be effective in reducing teacher-, parent-, and child self-reported externalizing behavior problems at the end of intervention that had been implemented with intensive training to "real-world" guidance counselors in schools (Lochman et al., 2009).

Case Example

Joshua, a 4th grader at Wilson Elementary School, has had behavior difficulties since he was a toddler. He was dismissed from two preschools for aggression toward other children and for not sitting still or following directions. At the time, Joshua's mother attributed his behavior problems to not having a father figure in his life. His biological father died of a drug overdose when Joshua was 4 years old. Joshua did not appear to be very affected by this loss, as he had had infrequent contact with his father before his death. Joshua's new stepfather has been in his life for several years now, and appears to be a positive influence on Joshua.

When Joshua began to struggle academically and behaviorally at school, his mother requested psychological testing. The assessment revealed that Joshua met diagnostic criteria for Attention-Deficit/Hyperactivity Disorder, Hyperactive/Impulsive Type (ADHD) and ODD. Through the evaluation process, Joshua's mother learned that Joshua's father and several of his paternal family members had been diagnosed with ADHD. At the end of 3rd grade, Joshua began taking stimulant medication. Joshua's academic performance improved, but he still had trouble following the teacher's directions and getting along with his peers. His mother sought a Section 504 plan so that Joshua would receive behavioral intervention at school.

The school psychologist, Dr. Carlisle, invited Joshua to join a small group that met weekly to provide social and emotional skills training for students with disruptive behavior problems (using the Coping Power curriculum). The group members first learned about setting personal behavior goals. With input from his mother and teacher, Joshua set a goal of taking time to calm down before reacting when something happened that made him angry. Dr. Carlisle asked Joshua's teacher to remind Joshua to use this strategy whenever she noticed him becoming angry in class and to give him positive feedback whenever he made an effort to do so. Joshua was proud to tell the other Coping Power group members that his teacher had given him a positive report on his goal sheet several days in a row.

In the next Coping Power unit, Joshua learned to recognize the early "clues" that his body gave him that he was starting to become angry (e.g., tense muscles, feeling hot). He also started to recognize situations in which he tended to feel this way (e.g., when he did not get his way). He learned to use self-calming strategies (e.g., deep breathing and coping self-statements, such as "don't be a fool, stay cool") that helped him create space between his angry feelings and his response to the situation. In the next unit, Joshua also learned to take time to see the situation from the other person's perspective (e.g., to think about why his mother may have told him that he could not do something he wanted to do), which led him to be less quick to lash out in anger.

Next, Joshua and the other group members learned to brainstorm solutions to social problems. At first, Joshua believed strongly that it is best to "show others they can't mess with you, even if it means fighting them." However, as the group learned about short-term and long-term consequences, Joshua realized that continuing to use this approach could make it difficult for him to reach his personal goals (e.g., to play on his school's basketball team). He and the other group members practiced alternative solutions to social problems (e.g., ignoring, assertive communication) and observed how these solutions tended to lead to better outcomes. Finally, Joshua and the other group members learned about the importance of affiliating with positive peers and they practiced strategies for resisting peer pressure.

Dr. Carlisle kept Joshua's teacher and parents informed of what he was learning and how they could encourage Joshua to use the same strategies in class and at home. By the end of the program, Joshua's teacher noticed that he was somewhat slower to anger and much more willing to hear others out. Furthermore, Joshua's mother and stepfather noticed that he was more successful in his peer interactions and better at following directions at home. They had participated in some parent group sessions, in which they learned the importance of taking time to positively connect with Joshua, to make an effort to reinforce his positive behavior, to encourage his involvement in family decision-making, to supervise his peer relationships and after school activities closely, and to follow a consistent system for giving instructions and providing consequences for compliant or noncompliant behavior. Joshua responded well to these changes and family members were able to enjoy each other much more at home.

Take-Home Points

- Disruptive behavior problems often co-occur with poor academic functioning and lower levels of school connectedness.
- Risk factors for youth aggression can include biology and temperament, community and neighborhood features, family issues, peer relations, and social cognitive functioning.

- Assessment of conduct problems should include data from multiple informants and from multiple instruments.
- Evidence-based treatments designed for youth conduct problems include LifeSkills Training, The Incredible Years, and Coping Power.

Resources

- NASP Resources–Behavior Problems: http://www.nasponline.org/resources/listingb.aspx
- LifeSkills Training: www.lifeskillstraining.com
- The Incredible Years: incredibleyears.com
- Coping Power: www.copingpower.com

References

American Psychiatric Association (APA). (2013). *Diagnostic and statistical manual of mental disorders* (5th ed.) (DSM-5). Washington, DC: American Psychiatric Association.

Barry, C.T., Golmaryami, F.N., Rivera-Hudson, N., & Frick, P.J. (2013). Evidence-based assessment of conduct disorder: Current considerations and preparation for DSM-5. *Professional Psychology: Research and Practice, 44*(1), 56.

Barry, T.D., Dunlap, S., Lochman, J.E., & Wells, K.C. (2009). Inconsistent discipline as a mediator between maternal distress and aggression in boys. *Child and Family Behavior Therapy, 31*, 1–19.

Barth, J.M., Dunlap, S.T., Dane, H., Lochman, J.E., & Wells, K.C. (2004). Classroom environment influences on aggression, peer relations, and academic focus. *Journal of School Psychology, 42*, 115–133.

Botvin, G.J., & Griffin, K.W. (2004). Life skills training: Empirical findings and future directions. *Journal of Primary Prevention, 25*(2), 211–232.

Botvin, G.J., & Kantor, L.W. (2000). Preventing alcohol and tobacco use through life skills training. *Alcohol Research And Health, 24*(4), 250–257.

Bowers, A.J. (2010). Grades and graduation: A longitudinal risk perspective to identify school dropouts. *The Journal of Educational Research, 103*, 191–207.

Bradshaw, C.P., Buckley, J., & Ialongo, N. (2008). School-based service utilization among urban children with early-onset educational and mental health problems: The squeaky wheel phenomenon. *School Psychology Quarterly, 23*, 169–186.

De Los Reyes, A., Henry, D.B., Tolan, P.H., & Wakschlag, L.S. (2009). Linking informant discrepancies to observed variations in young children's disruptive behavior. *Journal of Abnormal Child Psychology, 37*(5), 637–652.

Dishion, T.J., Andrews, D.W., & Crosby, L. (1995). Antisocial boys and their friends in early adolescence: Relationship characteristics, quality, and interactional process. *Child Development, 66*, 139–151.

Dodge, K.A., Lochman, J.E., Harnish, J.D., Bates, J.E., & Pettit, G.S. (1997). Reactive and proactive aggression in school children and psychiatrically impaired chronically assaultive youth. *Journal of Abnormal Psychology, 106*, 37–51.

Ellis, M.L., Weiss, B., & Lochman, J.E. (2009). Executive functions in children: Associations with aggressive behavior and social appraisal processing. *Journal of Abnormal Child Psychology, 37*, 945–956.

Essex, M.J., Kraemer, H.C., Slattery, M.J., Burk, L.R., Boyce, W., Woodward, H.R., & Kupfer, D.J. (2009). Screening for childhood mental health problems: Outcomes and early identification. *Journal of Child Psychology and Psychiatry, 50*(5), 562–570.

Fite, P.J., Wynn, P., Lochman, J.E., & Wells, K.C. (2009). The effect of neighborhood disadvantage on proactive and reactive aggression. *Journal of Community Psychology, 37*, 542–546.

Foley, D.L., Eaves, L.J., Wormley, B., Silberg, J.L., Maes, H.H., Kuhn, J., & Riley, B. (2004). Childhood adversity, monoamine oxidase A genotype, and risk for conduct disorder. *Archives of General Psychiatry, 61*, 738–744.

Frick, P.J., & Hare, R.D. (2001). *Antisocial process screening device: APSD*. Toronto: Multi-Health Systems.

Kazdin, A.E. (2005). Evidence-based assessment for children and adolescents: Issues in measurement development and clinical application. *Journal of Clinical Child and Adolescent Psychology, 34*(3), 548–558.

Lochman, J.E., Boxmeyer, C.L., & Powell, N.P. (2012). Cognitive-behavioral intervention for anger and aggression: The Coping Power Program. In S.R. Jimmerson, A.B. Nickerson, M.J. Mayer, & M.J. Furlong (Eds.), *Handbook of school violence and school safety: International research and practice* (2nd ed., pp. 579–591). New York, NY: Routledge.

Lochman, J.E., Boxmeyer, C., Powell, N., Qu, L., Wells, K., & Windle, M. (2009). Dissemination of the Coping Power program: Importance of intensity of counselor training. *Journal of Consulting and Clinical Psychology, 77*, 397–409.

Lochman, J.E., & Dodge, K.A. (1994). Social-cognitive processes of severely violent, moderately aggressive and nonaggressive boys. *Journal of Consulting and Clinical Psychology, 62*, 366–374.

Lochman, J.E., & Dodge, K.A. (1998). Distorted perceptions in dyadic interactions of aggressive and nonaggressive boys: Effects of prior expectations, context, and boys' age. *Development and Psychopathology, 10*, 495–512.

Lochman, J.E., FitzGerald, D.P., Gage, S.M., Kanaly, M.K., Whidby, J.M., Barry, T.D., . . . & McElroy, H. (2001). Effects of a social-cognitive intervention for aggressive deaf children: The Coping Power Program. *Journal of the American Deafness and Rehabilitation Association, 35*(2), 39–61.

Lochman, J.E., & Wayland, K.K. (1994). Aggression, social acceptance and race as predictors of negative adolescent outcomes. *Journal of the American Academy of Child and Adolescent Psychiatry, 33*, 1026–1035.

Lochman, J.E., Wayland, K.K., & White, K.J. (1993). Social goals: Relationship to adolescent adjustment and to social problem solving. *Journal of Abnormal Child Psychology, 21*, 135–151.

Lochman, J.E., & Wells, K.C. (2002a). Contextual social-cognitive mediators and child outcome: A test of the theoretical model in the Coping Power Program. *Development and Psychopathology, 14*, 971–993.

Lochman, J.E., & Wells, K.C. (2002b). The Coping Power Program at the middle school transition: Universal and indicated prevention effects. *Psychology of Addictive Behaviors, 16*, S40–S54.

Lochman, J.E., & Wells, K.C. (2003). Effectiveness study of Coping Power and classroom intervention with aggressive children: Outcomes at a one-year follow-up. *Behavior Therapy, 34*, 493–515.

Lochman, J.E., & Wells, K.C. (2004). The Coping Power program for preadolescent aggressive boys and their parents: Outcome effects at the one-year follow-up. *Journal of Consulting and Clinical Psychology, 72*, 571–578.

Lochman, J.E., Wells, K.C., Qu, L., & Chen, L. (2013). Three year follow-up of Coping Power intervention effects: Evidence of neighborhood moderation? *Prevention Science, 14*, 364-376.

Masten, A.S., Desjardins, C., McCormick, C.M., Kuo, S., & Long, J.D. (2010). The significance of childhood competence and problems for adult success in work: A developmental cascade analysis. *Development and Psychopathology, 22*(3), 679–694.

Matthys, W., & Lochman, J.E. (2010). *Oppositional Defiant Disorder and Conduct Disorder in children*. Oxford, England: Wiley-Blackwell.

Nock, M.K., Kazdin, A.E., Hiripi, E., & Kessler, R.C. (2007). Lifetime prevalence, correlates, and persistence of Oppositional Defiant Disorder: results from the National Comorbidity Survey Replication. *Journal of Child Psychology and Psychiatry, 48*(7), 703–713.

Orobio de Castro, B., Veerman, J.W., Koops, W., Bosch, J.D., & Monshouwer, H.J. (2002). Hostile attribution of intent and aggressive behavior: A meta-analysis. *Child Development, 73*(3), 916–934.

Pardini, D.A., Lochman, J.E., & Frick, P.J. (2003). Callous/unemotional traits and social cognitive processes in adjudicated youth. *Journal of the American Academy of Child and Adolescent Psychiatry, 42*, 364–371.

Reid, J.B., Patterson, G.R., & Snyder, J. (2002). *Antisocial behavior in children and adolescents. A developmental analysis and model of intervention*. Washington, DC: American Psychological Association.

Reid, M.J., Webster-Stratton, C., & Hammond, M. (2007). Enhancing a classroom social competence and problem-solving curriculum by offering parent training to families of moderate-to high-risk elementary school children. *Journal of Clinical Child and Adolescent Psychology, 36*(4), 605–620.

Reynolds, C.R., & Kamphaus, R.W. (2004). *BASC-2: Behavior assessment system for children*. Circle Pines, MN: AGS Publishing.

Sattler, J.M. (2001). *Assessment of children: Cognitive applications* (4th ed.). J.M. Sattler.

Shaffer, D., Fisher, P., Lucas, C.P., Dulcan, M.K., & Schwab-Stone, M.E. (2000). NIMH Diagnostic Interview Schedule for Children Version IV (NIMH DISC-IV): Description, differences from previous versions, and reliability of some common diagnoses. *Journal of the American Academy of Child & Adolescent Psychiatry, 39*(1), 28–38.

Smith, S.W., Lochman, J.E., & Daunic, A.P. (2005). Managing aggression using cognitive-behavioral interventions: State of the practice and future directions. *Behavioral Disorders, 30*, 227–240.

Thomas, D.E., Bierman, K.L., Thompson, C., Powers, C.J., & Conduct Problems Prevention Research Group. (2008). Double jeopardy: Child and school characteristics that predict aggressive-disruptive behavior in the first grade. *School Psychology Review, 37*, 516–532.

U.S. Department of Education. (2007). *27th annual report to Congress on the implementation of the Individuals with Disabilities Education Act, 2005* (Vol. 2). Washington, DC: Author.

van de Wiel, N.M.H., Matthys, W., Cohen-Kettenis, P.T., Maassen, G.H., Lochman, J.E., & van Engeland, H. (2007). The effectiveness of an experimental treatment when compared with care as usual depends on the type of care as usual. *Behavior Modification, 31*, 298–312.

Wagner, M., Newman, L., Cameto, R., & Levine, P. (2006). *The academic achievement andfunctional performance of youth with disabilities: Report from the National LongitudinalTransition Study—2 (NLST2). (NCSER 2006–3000)*. Menlo Park, CA: SRT International.

Wakschlag, L.S., Pickett, K.E., Kasza, K.E., & Loeber, R. (2006). Is prenatal smoking associated with a developmental pattern of conduct problems in young boys? *Journal of the American Academy of Child and Adolescent Psychiatry, 45*, 461–467.

Webster-Stratton, C., & Hammond, M. (1997). Treating children with early-onset conduct problems: A comparison of child and parent training interventions. *Journal of Consulting and Clinical Psychology, 65*, 93–109.

Webster-Stratton, C., & Reid, M. (2003). The Incredible Years parents, teachers and children training series: A multifaceted treatment approach for young children with conduct problems. In A.E. Kazdin & J.R. Weisz (Eds.), *Evidence-based psychotherapies for children and adolescents* (pp. 224–240). New York, NY: Guilford Press.

Webster-Stratton, C., & Reid, M. (2007). Incredible Years Parents and Teachers Training Series: A Head Start partnership to promote social competence and prevent conduct problems. In P. Tolan, J. Szapocznik, & S. Sambrano (Eds.), *Preventing youth substance abuse: Science-based programs for children and adolescents* (pp. 67–88). Washington, DC: American Psychological Association.

Webster-Stratton, C., Reid, M., & Hammond, M. (2001). Social skills and problem-solving training for children with early-onset conduct problems: Who benefits? *Journal of Child Psychology and Psychiatry, 42*, 943–952.

Webster-Stratton, C., Reid, M., & Hammond, M. (2004). Treating children with early-onset conduct problems: Intervention outcomes for parent, child, and teacher training. *Journal of Clinical Child and Adolescent Psychology, 33*, 105–124.

Williams, S.C., Lochman, J.E., Phillips, N.C., & Barry, T. (2003). Aggressive and nonaggressive boys' physiological and cognitive processes in response to peer provocations. *Journal of Clinical Child and Adolescent Psychology, 32*, 568–576.

3

INTERNALIZING BEHAVIORS

Janay B. Sander, Kimberly DeBoth, and Thomas H. Ollendick

Internalizing disorders refer primarily to anxiety and depressive disorders (Ollendick & Sander, 2012). In the most recent version of the DSM-5, seven distinct anxiety disorders are included: generalized anxiety disorder (GAD), separation anxiety disorder (SAD), social anxiety disorder (social phobia), specific phobia, selective mutism, agoraphobia, and panic disorder. Depressive disorders include disruptive mood dysregulation disorder (DMDD), which is a new diagnosis in the DSM-5, along with major depressive disorder (MDD), persistent depressive disorder, and premenstrual dysphoric disorder. For the anxiety and depressive disorders, "other," "unspecified," or "due to medical conditions" categories also exist (American Psychiatric Association, 2013).

There is a physiological, a cognitive, and a behavioral component to internalizing disorders. With anxiety disorders, there is a combination of anticipatory worry, physiological arousal symptoms of anxiety or fear, and behavioral avoidance. These symptoms are out of proportion to any actual threat or danger, so cognitively the threat is overestimated (APA, 2013). With depressive disorders, the irritable, hopeless, sad, or flat emotional experience is pervasive. There are accompanying physiologic changes in sleep, appetite, lethargic or agitated motor responses, and energy levels (APA, 2013). Common features include cognitive patterns of rumination over negative events and distortions about how events relate to the self (Hankin & Abramson, 2002). Externalizing problems and Autism Spectrum Disorders (ASD) may have overlapping symptoms with internalizing behaviors, including irritability, agitation, and inattention (Kendall, Settipani & Cummings, 2013).

DSM-5

There are several changes in the DSM-5 pertaining to internalizing problems. In the past, obsessive-compulsive disorders (OCD) and trauma-related disorders were considered internalizing disorders. OCD, characterized by intrusive thoughts, urges and/or repetitive and rigid behaviors that temporarily reduce anxiety, is now grouped with other similar disorders. This new section, obsessive-compulsive and related disorders, includes OCD, body dysmorphic disorder, hoarding, trichotillomania (hair pulling), and excoriation (skin-picking). Trauma-related disorders, which involve marked distress following a traumatic or highly stressful event, are also grouped in a separate section of the DSM-5. Those disorders that are no longer included in the anxiety or depressive disorders in DSM-5 will not be a focus of this chapter.

In the DSM-5 there are several updates within the anxiety and depressive disorders. First, there is the addition of selective mutism and separation anxiety disorder criteria acknowledging that those can be experienced by both adults and children (rather than classifying them as disorders of childhood alone). Next, the diagnosis of social phobia is now referred to as social anxiety disorder. The new diagnostic section elaborates on the symptoms of fear of evaluation or of experiencing humiliation and also includes criteria for children to experience fear with peers, not just with adults. A final significant change is the separation of agoraphobia from panic disorder. Previously, these were combined in panic disorder with agoraphobia, whereas in DSM-5 they are two separate disorders.

Another significant addition is the new diagnosis of disruptive mood dysregulation disorder (DMDD). DMDD has clear implications for school-based mental health. This diagnosis can only be applied to children and adolescents between 7 and 18 years. The key feature is persistent, chronic irritability, combined with temper outbursts usually initiated by the emotion of frustration. This is the only one of the depressive disorders that is more common in males than females. With DMDD as a diagnosis, what would have been considered a disruptive behavior disorder rather than a mood disorder may change perceptions and potentially allow for more services to be offered.

Prevalence

In the general population, between 10 and 15% of children and adolescents meet diagnostic criteria for an anxiety or depressive disorder at any given point in time (Ghandour, Kogan, Blumberg, Jones & Perrin, 2012). Major depression is a common disorder in the general population, and lifetime prevalence rates are approximately 17% (Kessler et al, 2005). Lifetime prevalence rates for anxiety disorders approach 25% by early adulthood (Copeland, Angold, Shanahan & Costello, 2014). In childhood, point prevalence rates for boys and girls for anxiety and depressive disorders is roughly 8% (Ghandour et al., 2012). These rates increase during adolescence for boys and girls. Beginning in early adolescence, girls' prevalence rates surpass those for boys for depressive disorders, reaching a 2:1 ratio (Orton, Riggs, & Libby, 2009). In subgroups in the population, such as low income groups, up to 17% of adolescent girls meet criteria for a depressive disorder, in contrast to 7% of boys in a similar subgroup (Orton et al., 2009). In special education subgroups in the school-age population, rates of anxiety or depressive disorders range from about 14% (Déry, Toupin, Pauzé, & Verlaan, 2004) to as high as 30% (Emerson, 2003).

Etiology

Although a definitive etiological pathway has not yet emerged, current research indicates that internalizing problems arise due to a combination of genetic, environmental (Nivard et al., 2015), personality, and cognitive factors within a diathesis-stress framework (Brozina & Abela, 2006; Hudson & Rapee, 2009). The overlap in anxiety and depression leads to a hypothesis about shared etiology (Mathew, Pettit, Lewinsohn, Seeley, & Roberts, 2011). At the same time, there is not consistent empirical support for a shared etiology across anxiety and depression (Ollendick, Grills, & Alexander, 2001).

Assessment

Best practices in assessment of internalizing disorders necessitates using multiple informants, such as parent report, observations, teacher report, and self report information whenever possible (McLeod, Jensen-Doss, & Ollendick, 2013). The use of a full diagnostic interview is not always feasible in a school setting, nor necessary, so the focus here is on the most efficient ways to measure symptoms that fit with school constraints. For internalizing disorders, there is generally poor agreement in ratings of adults and self-ratings by children and adolescents, even for children reporting elevated anxiety symptoms (Miller, Martinez, Shumka, & Baker, 2014). It is unclear why exactly that is the case, but use of clinical judgment in addition to ratings from multiple sources is necessary to accurately identify the children suffering from internalizing disorders.

We offer a general overview of assessment tools here. Other sources provide a more comprehensive review of evidence-based assessments of internalizing disorders (see Grills-Taquechel & Ollendick, 2012; McLeod et al., 2013). In brief, in a school setting there may be multiple purposes for using assessment: screening, diagnosis, and progress monitoring during intervention. In schools, the use of norm-referenced measures, with high reliability and validity, that include parent, teacher, and self report, is highly recommended (Maag & Swearer, 2005). For screening purposes, norm-referenced, brief rating tools that address anxiety and depressive symptoms include the Behavioral and Emotional Screening System (BESS), a short form of the more comprehensive rating tool with items to assess internalizing and externalizing concerns, the Behavioral Assessment System for Children, 2nd edition (BASC-2; Reynolds & Kamphaus, 2004). Another option is the Child Behavior Checklist (CBCL; Achenbach & Rescorla, 2001). These measures include self-, parent-, and teacher-report forms across internalizing and externalizing symptoms. For a symptom checklist, the Mood and Feelings

Questionnaire, developed by Angold, Costello, Messer and Pickles (1995), is a tool that has been used in several research projects and is available for download (see resources section at the conclusion of this chapter).

There are several self-report rating scales that can be used to screen for anxiety or depressive symptoms. These measures can also be used periodically to track progress in treatment and are fairly brief to administer. First, the Screen for Child Anxiety Related Disorders (SCARED) is a clinical self-report measure used for screening anxiety in children (Birmaher et al., 1999; see resources list at the conclusion of this chapter), and the developers have made this instrument available at no cost. Next, the Multidimensional Anxiety Scale for Children, Second Edition (MASC-2; March, 2012) is a commonly used anxiety rating scale that has good overall psychometric properties. Another option would be the Beck Youth Inventories, 2nd edition (BYI-II), the Anxiety and Depression Scales, which are reliable, valid, and intended to assess internalizing problems (Beck, Beck, & Jolly, 2005).

Lastly, behavioral observations in the school setting are often helpful. If a student is being evaluated for special education due to emotional issues, a functional behavioral assessment would typically be conducted. Furthermore, baseline observations would inform specific objectives and methods for measuring progress toward behavioral goals for special education students. In closing, whenever internalizing problems are identified in schools, we recommend using an objective, multiple-informant method to document level of impairment. That data should be linked with the intervention.

Evidence-based Interventions and Prevention

There are several evidence-based interventions for internalizing concerns (Ollendick & King, 2012). First, to treat anxiety, the following elements are associated with most gains in treatment: exposure, modeling, and information processing/cognitive change (Grills-Taquechel & Ollendick, 2012). The exposure component would occur in a graduated manner, and would include coping and relaxation training to help prepare the student for graduated exposures to the feared object or situation. Live exposure, *in vivo*, is preferable to imagined exposure. Modeling is the second element, which also has graduated components of increasing exposure and direct contact with the feared object or situation. Modeling can occur via video or in vivo in the presence of the child, coaching the child to interact with the feared object or situation. As an additional consideration, including rewards for interacting with a feared object or situation or at least for preventing escape or avoidance, is recommended for anxiety treatments. Individual formats are currently more supported than group interventions for anxiety disorders, specifically, but this area and also the role of parental involvement in treatment warrant further research (Ollendick & King, 2012).

School-based intervention programs that have been empirically tested to address anxiety include the FRIENDS program (Lowry-Webster, Barrett, &

Dadds, 2001), Cool Kids (Hudson, Lyneham, & Rapee, 2008), and Skills for Social and Academic Success (SASS) (Fisher, Masia-Warner, & Klein, 2004; Masia-Warner, Fisher, Shrout, Rathor, & Klein, 2007). The FRIENDS program is a brief intervention that can be implemented in groups or individually. The program includes relaxation techniques and coping, problem-solving skills, and exposure, and it has family and peer components (Barrett, Farrell, Ollendick, & Dadds, 2006). The Cool Kids program incorporates common elements in treating anxiety: psychoeducation, exposure, identification and modification of cognitive errors (see McLoone, Hudson, & Rapee, 2006). The SASS intervention is designed for social phobia, specifically, and includes elements of psychoeducation, skills training, exposure, modifying thinking errors, and use of peer assistants (Masia-Warner et al., 2007).

For depression, there are several manualized interventions with empirical support. These interventions include similar components of cognitive restructuring; psychoeducation about the symptoms and disorder; and affective education, problem-solving, and activity scheduling (Chorpita & Daleiden, 2009). First, the Coping with Depression for Adolescents (CWD-A) course (see resources section at the conclusion of this chapter) has been used in several outcome studies (see Clarke, Lewinsohn, & Hops, 1990). The Primary and Secondary Control Enhancement Training (PASCET) is another set of materials available from the authors to assist with teaching coping, behavioral activation, problem-solving, and cognitive restructuring for internalizing disorders (Weisz, Gray, Bearman, Southam-Gerow, & Stark, 2005). The Modular Approach to Therapy for Children with Anxiety, Depression, Trauma, and Conduct Problems (MATCH-ADTC) developed by Chorpita and Weisz (2009) is recommended for comorbid concerns in particular. The ACTION program is another option, which was developed for use in schools with adolescent girls (Stark et al., 2006).

Academic Implications

At times, teachers may not notice a student who experiences an internalizing disorder that does not include some externalizing symptoms. Typically, the worry, sadness, or fear would not necessarily be apparent, unless the student shares these feelings in writing or out loud. School staff may become aware of a problem if the student is frequently absent from school—a sign of school refusal that is often related to anxiety (Kearney, 2008). The school atmosphere, in itself, can be stress inducing. Students with anxiety disorders or sub-clinical symptoms of anxiety may have difficulty functioning in school (Mychailyszyn, Mendez, & Kendall, 2010; Schoenfeld & Janney, 2008).

Youth with anxiety related disorders, such as generalized anxiety disorder or social anxiety disorder, commonly worry regarding their performance at school (Mychailyszyn et al., 2010). Excessive worrying can affect students' test-taking ability, social relationships, behaviors, working memory, and attention

(Grills-Taquechel, Fletcher, Vaughn, Denton, & Taylor, 2013; Owens, Stevenson, Hadwin, & Norgate, 2012). Students may complain of somatic symptoms in order to avoid stress-invoking situations at school (Hughes, Lourea-Waddell, & Kendall, 2008).

Students with anxiety disorders may be impaired enough to receive special education services because of the impact of their anxiety symptoms on academic functioning (Schoenfeld & Janney, 2008). However, and unfortunately, it is uncommon for schools to provide interventions for students who have anxiety difficulties alone, without concurrent behavioral concerns. As a result, students may be significantly under-identified in terms of impairment caused by anxiety. Therefore, it is recommended that school personnel become aware of the possible academic challenges that may be faced by students with anxiety.

Similar to anxiety, symptoms of depression have negative cognitive and emotional complications that can significantly affect functioning in school (Owens et al., 2012). As such, depressive disorders have a clear impact on academic performance. Symptoms of depression as well as low self-efficacy are related to increased risk for dropping out of school (Quiroga, Janosz, Bisset, & Morin, 2013) and for lower grade point averages (Shahar et al., 2006). Adolescents with depression are also at particular risk for suicide (Rohde, Beevers, Stice, & O'Neil, 2009) and for dropping out of school before high school graduation (Quiroga et al., 2013).

Depression, or sad mood, is a documented area to consider for special education and related services under the eligibility category of emotional disturbance if there is demonstrated educational need. Federal regulations of the Individuals with Disabilities Education Act (IDEA), 20 United States Code § 1400 (2004), Part A Sec. 300.8 (c) (4) (i) include the words "pervasive mood of unhappiness or depression" in the definition of an emotional disturbance. This is important for school mental health practitioners to keep in mind, as it may indicate the need to advocate for appropriate services, including counseling or behavioral interventions and support for a student with internalizing problems who is receiving special education due to an emotional disability.

Furthermore, specific populations such as lesbian, gay, bisexual, and transgender (LGBT) students as well as victims of bullying are at high risk for developing symptoms of depression and anxiety (Herman, Reinke, Parkin, Traylor, & Agarwal, 2009). The range of emotional and cognitive symptoms of depression affects students' ability to complete work, interact with peers, and maintain attention at school.

Ethnic and Cultural Considerations

Ethnic and cultural factors are crucial to consider for both assessment and intervention. Common practice involves assessing symptoms by comparing age- and gender-based normative symptoms and behavior, but cultural and ethnic identity norms need to be considered as well (Cooley & Boyce, 2004; Oswald & Mazefsky,

2006). When providing interventions, it is always important to consider cultural factors. As an example, school-based cognitive behavioral therapy (CBT) has been recommended for a wide variety of clients from diverse backgrounds, including Filipino, East Indian, Asian and Hispanic adolescents, and has been effective in reducing symptoms (Manassis et al., 2010). When selecting interventions, clinicians should be aware of additional culturally based stressors that may be impeding functioning for clients, as well as culturally oriented strengths that may boost resilience. Specifically, clients may be experiencing acculturation stress as a result of transitioning to a majority culture (Cooley & Boyce, 2004). They may also draw upon social support or extended family, including formal and informal kinship, beyond the parent system (Jones, 2012).

Many interventions have been adapted for clients from diverse backgrounds, but the large body of research may not always reflect this in the randomized control trials. For clients of color experiencing depression or anxiety, for example, it would be important to remember that some negative experiences and fears are real concerns, not distorted exaggerations of social judgment or discrimination (Graham, Sorenson, & Hayes-Skelton, 2013). In schools, specifically, attending to culture, connections to families, school climate, and ongoing development of the clinician's cultural competence would relate to the client's engagement and the success of an intervention (Jones, 2012).

Case Illustration: Javier

Javier was a 13-year-old male in 7th grade who lived with his mother, step-father, and younger brother. Javier is Latino, of Mexican origin. His mother came to the United States as a teenager and Javier was born in the United States. He was referred for counseling at school by his mother, who was worried about him and thought he might be depressed. His father, deceased, had a history of depression, and so did his mother. The psychologist on staff at the school interviewed the parent, student, and teacher, conducted a classroom observation, and had parent, teacher, and Javier complete BASC-2 rating forms about his emotions and behaviors.

The teacher rating form indicated school learning concerns but was within the average range for depression and anxiety. Somatization was elevated. On the parent rating form, the scores on depression and anxiety scales were elevated. On the self-rating form, Javier reported elevated symptoms in the areas of school problems, internalizing problems, and attention problems. During the classroom observation, Javier appeared somewhat lethargic, sat quietly, and did not actively participate in the class discussion. He was sitting in the front row and had his class materials open. The teacher called on him once to answer a question and Javier only replied, "I don't know," then looked down at his desk. In a diagnostic symptom interview, conducted with Javier and his mother separately, Javier met criteria for Persistent Depressive Disorder. Javier also conveyed how much he felt like a failure, and that he was always disappointed in himself for not doing better in school, even when he tried his best.

The psychologist began providing CBT at school to Javier, and also met with teachers individually (with appropriate consent) in order to boost positive classroom experiences and ensure some academic success would be possible for Javier. The teachers admitted they had assumed Javier was just "lazy," but became more sympathetic after learning more about childhood depression, Javier's background, and how much Javier genuinely wanted to succeed in school.

Take-Home Points

- Internalizing problems frequently overlap with externalizing problems.
- Internalizing problems often go unrecognized in school settings.
- Assessment tools for internalizing problems are used in the school setting.
- There are several evidence-based interventions for internalizing problems that have been used in school settings.

Resources

Helpful websites for no-cost downloads:

- Mood and Feelings Questionnaire: http://devepi.duhs.duke.edu/mfq.html
- SCARED Assessment: http://psychiatry.pitt.edu/research/tools-research
- Coping with Depression for Adolescents Course: http://www.kpchr.org/research/public/acwd/acwd.html

References

Achenbach, T.M., & Rescorla, L.A. (2001). *Manual for the ASEBA school-age forms and profiles*. Burlington, VT: University of Vermont.

American Psychiatric Association (APA). (2013). *Diagnostic and statistical manual of mental disorders* (5th ed.) (DSM-5). Washington, DC: American Psychiatric Association.

Angold, A., Costello, E.J., Messer, S.C., & Pickles, A. (1995). Development of a short questionnaire for use in epidemiological studies of depression in children and adolescents. *International Journal of Methods In Psychiatric Research*, *5*(4), 237–249.

Barrett, P.M., Farrell, L.J., Ollendick, T.H., & Dadds, M. (2006). Long-term outcomes of an Australian universal prevention trial of anxiety and depression symptoms in children and youth: An evaluation of the Friends program. *Journal of Clinical Child and Adolescent Psychology*, *35*(3), 403–411.

Beck, J.S., Beck, A.T., & Jolly, J.B. (2005). *Beck Youth Inventories, 2nd ed.* San Antonio, TX: Psychological Corporation.

Birmaher, B., Brent, D.A., Chiapetta, L., Bridge, J., Monga, S., & Baugher, M. (1999). Psychometric properties of the Screen for Child Anxiety Related Emotional Disorders (SCARED): A replication study. *Journal of the American Academy of Child and Adolescent Psychiatry*, *38*(10), 1230–6.

Brozina, K., & Abela, J.R. (2006). Behavioural inhibition, anxious symptoms, and depressive symptoms: A short-term prospective examination of a diathesis-stress model. *Behaviour Research and Therapy, 44*(9), 1137–1346.

Chorpita, B.F., & Daleiden, E.L. (2009). Mapping evidence-based treatments for children and adolescents: Application of the distillation and matching model to 615 treatments from 322 randomized trials. *Journal of Consulting and Clinical Psychology*, 77(3), 566–579. doi: 10.1037/a0014565

Chorpita, B.F., & Weisz, J.R. (2009). *Modular approach to therapy for children with anxiety, depression, trauma, or conduct problems (MATCH-ADTC)*. Satellite Beach, FL: Practicewise, LLC

Clarke, G.N., Lewinsohn, P.M., & Hops, H. (1990). *Adolescent coping with depression course*. Retrieved from http://www.kpchr. org/acwd/acwd.html

Cooley, M.R., & Boyce, C.A. (2004). An introduction to assessing anxiety in child and adolescent multiethnic populations: Challenges and opportunities for enhancing knowledge and practice. *Journal of Clinical Child and Adolescent Psychology, 33*(2), 210–215. doi: 10.1207/s15374424jccp3302_1

Copeland, W.E., Angold, A., Shanahan, L., & Costello, E. (2014). Longitudinal patterns of anxiety from childhood to adulthood: The Great Smoky Mountains study. *Journal of the American Academy of Child & Adolescent Psychiatry, 53*(1), 21–33. doi: 10.1016/j.jaac.2013.09.017

Déry, M., Toupin, J., Pauzé, R., & Verlaan, P. (2004). Frequency of mental health disorders in a sample of elementary school students receiving special educational services for behavioural difficulties. *The Canadian Journal of Psychiatry / La Revue Canadienne De Psychiatrie, 49*(11), 769–775.

Emerson, E. (2003). Prevalence of psychiatric disorders in children and adolescents with and without intellectual disability. *Journal of Intellectual Disability Research, 47*, 51–58. doi: 10.1046/j.1365–2788.2003.00464.x

Fisher, P.H., Masia-Warner, C., & Klein, R.G. (2004). Skills for social and academic success: A school-based intervention for social anxiety disorder in adolescents. *Clinical Child and Family Psychology Review*, 7(4), 241–249. doi: 10.1007/s10567–004–6088–7

Ghandour, R.M., Kogan, M.D., Blumberg, S.J., Jones, J.R., & Perrin, J.M. (2012). Mental health conditions among school-aged children: Geographic and sociodemographic patterns in prevalence and treatment. *Journal of Developmental and Behavioral Pediatrics, 33*(1), 42–54. doi: 10.1097/DBP.0b013e31823e18fd

Graham, J.R., Sorenson, S., & Hayes-Skelton, S.A. (2013). Enhancing the cultural sensitivity of cognitive behavioral interventions for anxiety in diverse populations. *The Behavior Therapist, 36*(5), 101–108.

Grills-Taquechel, A.E., Fletcher, J.M., Vaughn, S.R., Denton, C.A., & Taylor, P. (2013). Anxiety and inattention as predictors of achievement in early elementary school children. *Anxiety, Stress & Coping: An International Journal, 26*(4), 391–410.

Grills-Taquechel, A.E., & Ollendick, T.H. (2012). *Phobic and anxiety disorders in youth*. Cambridge, MA: Hogrefe & Huber Publishers.

Hankin, B.L., & Abramson, L.Y. (2002). Measuring cognitive vulnerability to depression in adolescence: Reliability, validity, and gender differences. *Journal of Clinical Child and Adolescent Psychology, 31*(4), 491–504.

Herman, K.C., Reinke, W.M., Parkin, J., Traylor, K.B., & Agarwal, G. (2009). Childhood depression: Rethinking the role of the school. *Psychology in the Schools, 46*(5), 433–446.

Hudson, J.L., Lyneham, H.J., & Rapee, R.M. (2008). Social anxiety. In A.R. Eisen & A.R. Eisen (Eds.), *Treating childhood behavioral and emotional problems: A step-by-step evidence-based approach* (pp. 53–101). New York, NY: Guilford Press.

Hudson, J.L., & Rapee, R.M. (2009). Familial and social environments in the etiology and maintenance of anxiety disorders. In M.M. Antony, M.B. Stein, M.M. Antony, & M.B. Stein (Eds.), *Oxford handbook of anxiety and related disorders* (pp. 173–189). New York, NY: Oxford University Press.

Hughes, A.A., Lourea-Waddell, B., & Kendall, P.C. (2008). Somatic complaints in children with anxiety disorders and their unique prediction of poorer academic performance. *Child Psychiatry and Human Development, 39*(2), 211–220.

Jones, J.M. (2012). Family, school and community partnerships. In D. Shriberg, S.Y. Song, A.H. Miranda, & K.M. Radliff (Eds.), *School psychology and social justice: Conceptual foundations and tools for practice* (pp. 270–293). New York: Routledge Press.

Kearney, C.A. (2008). *Helping school refusing children and their parents: A guide for school-based professionals.* New York, NY: Oxford University Press.

Kendall, P.C., Settipani, C.A., & Cummings, C.M. (2013). No need to worry: The promising future of child anxiety research. *Journal of Clinical Child and Adolescent Psychology, 41*, 103–115.

Kessler, R.C., Berglund, P., Demler, O., Jin, R., Merikangas, K.R., & Walters, K.R. (2005). Lifetime prevalence and age-of-onset distributions of DSM-IV disorders in the national comorbidity survey replication. *Archives of General Psychiatry, 62*, 593–602.

Lowry-Webster, H.M., Barrett, P.M., & Dadds, M.R. (2001). A universal prevention trial of anxiety and depressive symptomatology in childhood: Preliminary data from an Australian study. *Behaviour Change, 18*(1), 36–50. doi: 10.1375/bech.18.1.36

Maag, J.W., & Swearer, S.M. (2005). Cognitive-behavioral interventions for depression: Review and implications for school personnel. *Behavioral Disorders, 30*(3), 259–276.

Manassis, K., Wilansky-Traynor, P., Farzan, N., Kleiman, V., Parker, K., & Sanford, M. (2010). The feelings club: Randomized controlled evaluation of school-based CBT for anxious or depressive symptoms. *Depression and Anxiety, 27*(10), 945–952. doi: 10.1002/da.20724

March, J.S. (2012). *Multidimensional Anxiety Scale for Children, Second Edition.* North Tonawanda, NY: Multi-Health Systems Inc.

Masia-Warner, C., Fisher, P.H., Shrout, P.E., Rathor, S., & Klein, R.G. (2007). Treating adolescents with social anxiety disorder in school: An attention control trial. *Journal of Child Psychology and Psychiatry, 48*(7), 676–686.

Mathew, A.R., Pettit, J.W., Lewinsohn, P.M., Seeley, J.R., & Roberts, R.E. (2011). Co-morbidity between major depressive disorder and anxiety disorders: Shared etiology or direct causation?. *Psychological Medicine, 41*(10), 2023–2034. doi: 10.1017/S0033291711000407

McLeod, B.D., Jensen-Doss, A., & Ollendick, T.H. (2013). *Diagnostic and behavioral assessment in children and adolescents: A clinical guide.* New York, NY: Guilford Press.

McLoone, J., Hudson, J.L., & Rapee, R.M. (2006). Treating anxiety disorders in a school setting. *Education & Treatment Of Children, 29*(2), 219–242.

Miller, L.D., Martinez, Y.J., Shumka, E., & Baker, H. (2014). Multiple informant agreement of child, parent, and teacher ratings within community samples. *The Canadian Journal of Psychiatry / La Revue Canadienne De Psychiatrie, 59*(1), 34–39.

Mychailyszyn, M.P., Mendez, J.L., & Kendall, P.C. (2010). School functioning in youth with and without anxiety disorders: Comparisons by diagnosis and comorbidity. *School Psychology Review, 39*(1), 106–121.

Nivard, M.G., Dolan, C.V., Kendler, K.S., Kan, K., Willemsen, G., van Beijsterveldt, C.M., ... Boomsma, D.I. (2015). Stability in symptoms of anxiety and depression as a function of genotype and environment: a longitudinal twin study from ages 3 to 63 years. *Psychological Medicine, 45*(5), 1039–1049. doi: 10.1017/S003329171400213X

Ollendick, T.H., Grills, A.E., & Alexander, K.L. (2001). Fears, worries, and anxiety in children and adolescents. In C.A. Essau & F. Petermann (Eds.), *Anxiety disorders in children and adolescents: Epidemiology, risk factors and treatment* (pp. 1–35). New York, NY: Psychology Press.

Ollendick, T.H., & King, N.J. (2012). Evidence-based treatments for children and adolescents: Issues and controversies. In P.C. Kendall (Ed.), *Child and adolescent therapy: Cognitive-behavioral procedures* (pp. 499–519). New York: Guilford Publications.

Ollendick, T.H., & Sander, J.B. (2012). Internalizing disorders in children and adolescents. In J.E. Maddux & B.A. Winstead (Eds.), *Psychopathology: Foundations for a contemporary understanding* (pp. 473–498). Mahwah, NJ: Lawrence Erlbaum Associates.

Orton, H.D., Riggs, P.D., & Libby, A.M. (2009). Prevalence and characteristics of depression and substance use in a U.S. child welfare sample. *Children and Youth Services Review, 31*(6), 649–653. doi: 10.1016/j.childyouth.2008.12.005

Oswald, D.P., & Mazefsky, C.A. (2006). Empirically supported psychotherapy interventions for internalizing disorders. *Psychology in the Schools, 43*(4), 439–449. doi: 10.1002/pits.20158

Owens, M., Stevenson, J., Hadwin, J.A., & Norgate, R. (2012). Anxiety and depression in academic performance: An exploration of the mediating factors of worry and working memory. *School Psychology International, 33*(4), 433–449.

Quiroga, C.V., Janosz, M., Bisset, S., & Morin, A.S. (2013). Early adolescent depression symptoms and school dropout: Mediating processes involving self-reported academic competence and achievement. *Journal of Educational Psychology, 105*(2), 552–560.

Reynolds, C.R., & Kamphaus, R.W. (2004). *Manual for the Behavioral Assessment System for Children, 2nd edition.* AGS Publishing.

Rohde, P., Beevers, C.G., Stice, E., & O'Neil, K. (2009). Major and minor depression in female adolescents: Onset, course, symptom presentation, and demographic associations. *Journal of Clinical Psychology, 65*(12), 1339–1349.

Schoenfeld, N.A., & Janney, D.M. (2008). Identification and treatment of anxiety in students with emotional or behavioral disorders: A review of the literature. *Education & Treatment Of Children, 31*(4), 583–610.

Shahar, G., Henrich, C.C., Winokur, A., Blatt, S.J., Kuperminc, G.P., & Leadbeater, B.J. (2006). Self-criticism and depressive symptomatology interact to predict middle school academic achievement. *Journal of Clinical Psychology, 62*(1), 147–155.

Stark, K.D., Hargrave, J., Sander, J., Custer, G., Schnoebelen, S., Simpson, J., & Molnar, J. (2006). Treatment of Childhood Depression: The ACTION Treatment Program. In P.C. Kendall & P.C. Kendall (Eds.), *Child and adolescent therapy: Cognitive-behavioral procedures* (3rd ed., pp. 169–216). New York, NY: Guilford Press.

Weisz, J.R., Gray, J.S., Bearman, S.K., Southam-Gerow, M., & Stark, K.D. (2005). *Primary and Secondary Control Enhancement Training Program: Therapists Manual (2nd ed.)*. Unpublished manuscript. Harvard University.

4

LEARNING DISABILITIES: ACADEMIC AND MENTAL HEALTH NEEDS

Elizabeth Swanson and Sharon Vaughn

Since 1874, when Carl Wernicke published ten case studies of "brain-injured" patients with language disorders (Wernicke, 1874), scientists have been intrigued with the phenomenon experienced by now more than 4.4 million children in the United States who are of at least average intellect, have no sensory disorders that would cause academic difficulty (e.g., blindness, deafness), but still struggle in learning and in life's daily demands. Samuel Kirk coined the term "learning disability" (LD) in his 1962 textbook, *Educating Exceptional Children*. He defined LD as follows:

> A retardation, disorder, or delayed development in one or more of the processes of speech, language, reading, writing, arithmetic, or other school subject resulting from a psychological handicap caused by a possible cerebral dysfunction and/or emotional or behavioral disturbances. It is not the result of mental retardation, sensory deprivation, or cultural and instructional factors (Kirk, 1962, p. 34).

A focus on specialized instruction for students with LD, begun in the 1920s, continued and was implemented in public schools beginning in 1975 (for a review of this history, see Hallahan, Pullen, & Ward, 2013). Diagnosticians have relied on the *Diagnostic and Statistical Manual of Mental Disorders* (DSM; American Psychiatric Association, 2013) to identify students with LD so that these individuals may access the services entitled to them in public schools. The newest DSM, the 5th edition, coupled with high quality research into intervention effects, now makes it possible to identify with a high degree of precision children, young adults, and adults who have LD and to subsequently manage the symptoms of LD with highly effective and proven treatments (Shaywitz, 2004). However, treatment almost exclusively involves academic interventions and rarely includes mental health services in spite of the fact that students with LD experience higher levels of anxiety and depression than their non-LD peers (Nelson & Harwood, 2011a; 2011b). In this chapter, we briefly review the DSM-5 LD diagnostic criteria, describe academic, social/emotional, and mental health difficulties students with LD often encounter, and propose ways in which taking the academic and mental health status of students with LD into account can influence practice and student outcomes.

Learning Disability Defined

DSM-5 definition. The DSM-5 provides clarified guidelines for identifying students with LD, reflecting changes in the Individuals with Disabilities Education Improvement Act of 2004 (IDEA; U.S. Department of Education, 2014) that broaden identification beyond the earlier standard IQ-achievement discrepancy formula. Instead, the new guidelines provide the mental health and education communities the opportunity to use a Response to Intervention (RTI) model as part of the identification process. It should be noted that using an RTI model as part of the identification process does not eliminate the requirement for a comprehensive evaluation (Fletcher, Steubing, Morris, & Lyon, 2013). Instead, it can now be used in conjunction.

Figure 4.1 provides a review of the new DSM-5 diagnostic criteria. In contrast to previous versions of the DSM that confined diagnosis to (a) reading disorder, (b) mathematics disorder, (c) disorder of written expression, or (d) learning disorder not otherwise specified, the categories are now more representative of the pervasive difficulties students with LD face across academic areas. Because prior classifications often overlapped and were highly interrelated (Tannock, 2013), the DSM-5 provides a unitary term that captures the overall difficulty experienced in academics. The learning disability category is now "Specific Learning Disorder." Using this overarching term, diagnosticians can then specify the details of the areas of difficulty as well as the severity (i.e., mild, moderate, or severe).

Prevalence and comorbidity. More than 4.4 million children in America are diagnosed with LD. Students with LD make up 40.1% of all school aged children identified with a disability, making LD the largest disability group in schools (U.S. Department of Education, 2014). Most students (67.2%) with LD are served in the general education setting for 80% or more of the school day (U.S. Department of Education, 2014). In 2012, a total of 68.8% of students with LD graduated with a regular high school diploma and, while the number of students with LD who drop out has decreased over the years, 19.9% of them dropped out of high school in 2012 (U.S. Department of Education, 2014).

LDs often occur in conjunction with other disorders or disabilities. For example, in a review (DuPaul, Gormley, & Laracy, 2013) of 17 studies investigating the comorbidity of Attention-Deficit/Hyperactivity Disorder (ADHD) and LD,

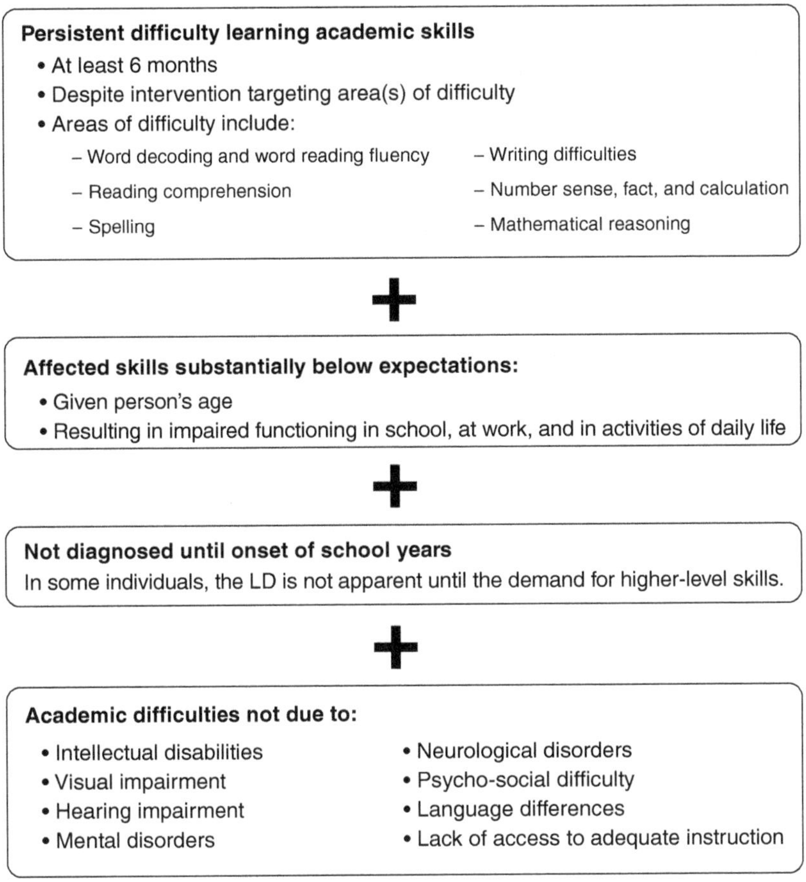

FIGURE 4.1 An outline of the DSM-5 diagnostic criteria for Specific Learning Disorder.

the authors determined that approximately 45.1% of students with ADHD were also diagnosed with an LD. Students with ADHD seem to be more likely to be co-diagnosed with a writing disability than a reading disability. LD in math is least often identified as comorbid with ADHD. For these reasons, a comprehensive assessment battery is essential when identifying a LD in school aged children.

Special considerations for English language learners (ELL). LD affects all subgroups of the U.S. population, no matter age, race, language background, or socioeconomic status. However, ELLs tend to be overrepresented in the LD category (Artiles & Ortiz, 2002). One reason for this trend may be the fact that ELLs are also often overlooked for early intervention in grades 1 and 2 (McCardle, Mele-McCarthy, Cutting, Leos, & Emilio, 2005), producing persistent unremediated difficulties (Lesaux & Harris, 2013). As a result, by 3rd grade ELLs may perform quite low on achievement tests. Therefore, it may be that waiting until

3rd grade or later and using discrepancy formulas for LD identification produces this over-identification problem. For ELLs in particular, a robust RTI program (described later in the chapter) that identifies academic difficulty early in the school career is essential for not only remediating difficulties early on, but also accurately identifying LD within the ELL population.

Academic Issues for Students with LD

As with all DSM-diagnosed disorders, there exists a spectrum of LD symptoms and severity. While some students may struggle with executive processing, others may struggle with language-based difficulties, and some students with LD experience deficits in both. Almost all students with LD experience some kind of social difficulty and have mental health needs associated with the academic and social emotional difficulties they encounter daily. In this section, we focus on academic issues for students and treating LD through RTI practices.

Executive processing. The span of executive processing skills includes coordination of memory systems, control of encoding and retrieval strategies, planning, switching attention when manipulating material, and retrieval of knowledge from long-term memory, among others. Within this set is working memory, which refers to processing resources of limited capacity that are involved in the preservation of information that is recalled and used simultaneously while learning new information (National Center for Learning Disabilities, 2014). Working memory is believed to be affected in a majority of students with LD; these students often exhibit (1) an inability to suppress irrelevant information and (2) difficulty with verbal and visual-spatial tasks that require simultaneous storage and processing (Swanson & Zheng, 2013). In an early study examining suppression of irrelevant information (Swanson & Cochran, 1991), students with and without LD were asked to listen to a list of words and remember as many as possible. Students without LD exhibited higher levels of recall than students with LD. Difficulty with simultaneous memory storage and processing manifests itself in "updating" what they know or have just learned (Miyake, Friedman, Emerson, Witzki, Howerter, & Wager, 2000). This updating requires (a) learning new information, (b) deciding its relevance to the task at hand, and then (c) revising information in working memory (Swanson & Zheng, 2013). In sum, students with LD exhibit more restricted working memory spans than students without LD, making it difficult for students with LD to suppress irrelevant information and update new knowledge as they learn.

Working memory difficulties manifest themselves in unique ways in the classroom. When writing, students may experience great difficulty engaging simultaneously in planning and organizing, composing, and editing for spelling and grammar, all the while remembering their audience and purpose for writing. The task of reading is at least equally complex. Not only are students required to remember letter names and, often, multiple associated phonemes, but they also must remember how these phonemes behave in combination. There are distractions in many words that make decoding difficult. Take the word "gnash" for example, in which one must remember that the "g" is silent—irrelevant information that students with LD may not be able to suppress. Reading comprehension can be particularly challenging. For example, a child may take a very long time to read a passage and, when finished, may say something like, "I don't really get what the book was about." Students with LD often experience difficulty identifying the main idea of a passage or cannot create a mental image of what is happening in the story. Picking out key facts from informational text may be difficult as well.

Another executive processing skill that causes difficulty for students with LD is Rapid Automatic Naming (RAN), defined as how quickly students can name continuously presented, highly familiar visual stimuli, such as digits, letters, or objects (Georgiou & Parrila, 2013). RAN has been reported as a strong predictor of academic outcomes (e.g., Lepola, Poskiparta, Laakkonen, & Niemi, 2005; Powell, Stainthorp, Stuart, Garwood, & Quinlan, 2007; Schatschneider, Fletcher, Francis, Carlson, & Foorman, 2004). While understood to be predictive of reading ability (e.g., Bowers, 2001; Powell et al., 2007), the processes underlying RAN are complex and multi-faceted: For example, while some students struggle with RAN skills such as phonological processing (i.e., rate of retrieval of letter sounds from long term memory; Torgesen, Wagner, & Rashotte, 1994), others have difficulty with orthographic processing (i.e., retrieving letter names when a symbol is seen on the page; Bowers & Wolf, 1993) or letter string identification (i.e., speed at which students identify letter strings as words; Bowers, 2001).

These same RAN-related difficulties interfere with mathematics learning as well. Take, for example, numeracy, wherein typically achieving students are able to determine the quantity of three or four objects without counting, can add and subtract small quantities to and from these sets, and understand concepts like "more" resulting from adding one item to a set (Case & Okamoto, 1996; Mandler & Shebo, 1982; Wynn, 1992; Wynn, Bloom & Chiang, 2002). Another example is counting, which is more complicated than it may seem to the informal observer and actually comprises at least three principles that mature during preschool years among typically achieving students: (a) one-to-one correspondence (i.e., one number word for each item); (b) stable order (i.e., number words are always in the same order), and (c) cardinality (i.e., last number word is the total in the set). Students with LD in mathematics may meet these developmental milestones later and may require explicit, remedial instruction to understand all of these principles. As students age, they may find arithmetic to be particularly difficult due to under-developed numeracy or principles of counting. Another explanation may be difficulties with working memory that prevent them from suppressing extra information or accessing prior numeracy knowledge when needed. RAN may pose a problem as well, preventing students with LD in mathematics from doing reading and calculations quickly enough to remember the goal of the mathematical task at hand.

Language-based difficulties. Of course, working memory and RAN are not the only explanatory variables that cause difficulties in school for students with LD. Language difficulties can also interfere with reading, writing, and/or math performance. While some students diagnosed with LD struggle with communication early in life, others experience differentially manifested language-related difficulties. Students with LD in reading, for example, may experience phonological deficits that interfere with developing phonological awareness and learning to decode (Goswami, 2002; Vellutino, Fletcher, Snowling & Scanlon, 2004; Georgiou & Parrila, 2013). For these students, learning letter names, their associated sounds, and the ways in which sounds work together to form words is exceedingly difficult and interferes with reading and understanding connected text. In other cases, phonological processing is intact but other language difficulties may be related to late-emerging or persistent LD in reading comprehension (Catts, Compton, Tomblin, & Bridges, 2012). Of course, etiology of LD is multifaceted and different students with LD may present with different symptoms. Even with the multifaceted nature of LD, important gains have been made in treating the symptoms of LD.

Treating LD Through RTI

RTI is a system-level, proactive, and preventative approach that relies on data-based decision-making to identify students who (a) are at risk for reading difficulty and (b) have an LD (Barnes & Harlacher, 2008; Fletcher & Vaughn, 2009). In this way, RTI has the potential to raise the achievement level of all students. Basically, students are identified for increasingly intensive intervention based on their low response to typically effective instructional practices. In this chapter, we will provide an overview of a three-tiered approach (a more complete explanation of a three-tiered RTI model may be found in Swanson & Vaughn, 2011). However, the number of tiers is not the most critical feature of RTI, as four- and even five-tiered approaches are used in schools (see Kovaleski & Black, 2010).

Generally speaking, within a three-tiered model, primary prevention of difficulty takes place in Tier 1, in which all students are provided research-based reading instruction in the general education classroom. Because no curriculum or methodology meets the needs of all students at all times, approximately 20% of students will require more intensive Tier 2 prevention in the form of supplemental intervention provided by the classroom teacher or a specialist. These short-term prevention programs are usually provided 3–5 days per week in small groups of 3–5 students over approximately 10 weeks in addition to effective Tier 1 intervention. One of two outcomes results from Tier 2 instruction. Either students meet grade-level expectations and Tier 2 intervention is discontinued, or students continue to experience difficulty. For these 2–3% of students, Tier 3 intervention that is more intensive, individualized, and provided in addition to Tier 1 instruction is necessary. Like Tier 2, Tier 3 instruction is delivered in small, homogeneous groups and consists of carefully designed, intensive, scientifically based reading instruction. However, the intensity of instruction and length of intervention sessions increases in Tier 3. A reading specialist or special education teacher who is well trained in the intervention usually delivers instruction. It is at this point that teachers and diagnosticians may consider the existence of an LD. Diagnosticians then take the lead in conducting a comprehensive assessment battery to inform decisions based on DSM-5 criteria. For more information about evidence-based interventions that are effective among students with LD, visit the Texas Center for Learning Disabilities at www.texasldcenter.org or the Building RTI Capacity website at www.buildingrti.utexas.org.

Social and Emotional Functioning and Mental Health Among Students with LD

Students with LD also experience social, emotional, and mental health issues. Special education teachers are not usually trained to deliver social or emotional interventions, meaning that most students with LD receive no intervention focused on these needs (Nelson & Harwood, 2011a; 2011b). However, mental health professionals are uniquely qualified to assist in these areas. Because social and emotional functioning and mental health are addressed at length elsewhere in this volume, we will focus on the ways in which students with LD are affected as well as special considerations required when diagnosing and treating students with LD for social and emotional functioning deficits or mental health needs.

Social and emotional functioning. While difficulties with social functioning alone do not constitute a learning disability, it is an area in which many students with LD struggle. A synthesis of 152 studies (Kavale & Forness, 1996) indicated that teachers report the social skills of students with LD are almost two-thirds of a standard deviation below those of typically achieving peers, meaning that almost three out of four students with LD would receive a more negative assessment of social skills (mean effect size = 0.65).

Adolescents with LD more often engage in externalizing behaviors, such as antisocial and aggressive behaviors, than do typically developing adolescents. Intrapersonal difficulties often plague students with LD as well, and these include anxiety, depression, withdrawn behaviors, and loneliness (Estell et al., 2008; Margalit, 2010). As with most manifestations of LD, there may be a multitude of reasons for these social issues, but for the sake of discussion they can be reduced to primary and/or secondary causes.

Primary causes of social emotional difficulties. The social information-processing (SIP) model (Crick & Dodge, 1994) provides some insight into the reasons students with LD may experience inter- and intra-personal difficulties in their daily lives. In this six-step model, many social-cognitive skills are required when navigating the social landscape (see Figure 4.2).

Students move from encoding and interpreting social cues to formulating a plan that meets their goal and, finally, determining whether the anticipated

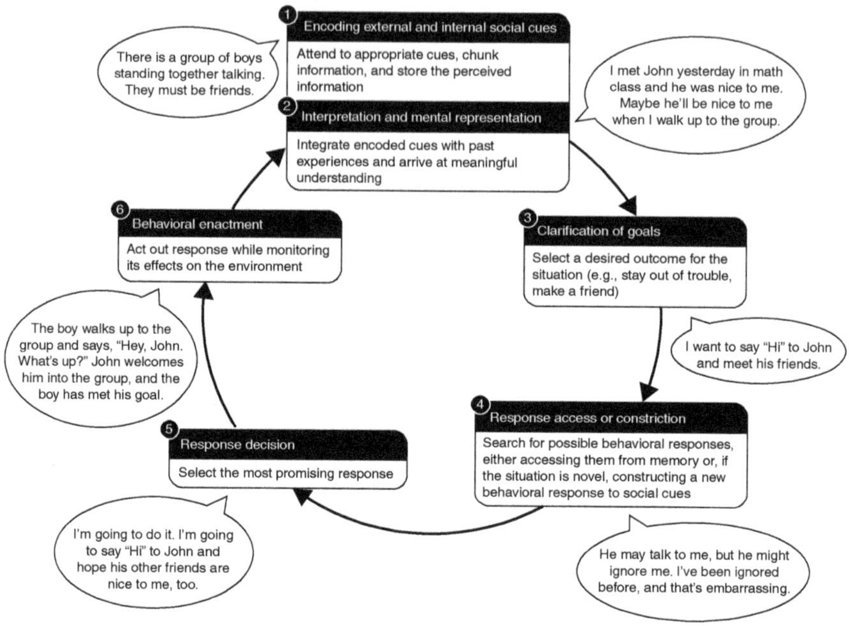

FIGURE 4.2 Six-step social information-processing (SIP) model (based on Crick & Dodge, 1994).

effect was achieved. There are many opportunities for students with LD who have working memory and language-based difficulties to make missteps along the way. They often misinterpret social situations. In a recent study (Galway & Metsala, 2011), students with language-based LD were less able to encode social cues and were less adept at interpreting those cues when compared to typically achieving peers. In addition, their problem solving skills are often impaired, leaving them less able to identify a social problem, generate alternative solutions, and accomplish desired social outcomes (Galway & Metsala, 2011; Toro, Weissberg, Guare, & Liebenstein, 1990).

Secondary causes of social emotional difficulties. Students with LD have a lower self-concept regarding their academic skills (Kavale & Forness, 1996; Tabassam & Grainger, 2002) compared to their non-LD peers. In fact, students with LD report their perceived academic competence as low, with an effect size of 0.95, indicating that more than eight out of ten students viewed themselves as deficient in academic skills. Similarly, lower reports exist of their nonverbal communication ability (ES = 0.94), social problem solving (ES = 0.90), social competence (ES = 0.80), self-concept (ES = .50), and self-esteem (ES = .42; Kavale & Forness, 1996). Indeed, students with LD are aware of their academic deficits, and this awareness seems to affect areas of social functioning; the secondary cause hypothesis is that academic self-concept is so low among students with LD due to school failure (Kloomok & Cosden, 1994) that it effects social functioning (Elbaum & Vaughn, 2003). These negative self-perceptions can be extremely difficult to change (Elbaum & Vaughn, 2003; Swann, 1996) and can range in severity from minimal to quite noticeable.

Mental health. Most of the work related to mental health and students with LD has focused on general anxiety. In a recent meta-analysis of 42 studies investigating the prevalence of anxiety among students with LD (Nelson & Harwood, 2011a), a moderate effect size was reported ($d = 0.61$), meaning that students with LD had higher mean scores on measures of anxiety than students without LD. In other words, approximately 70% of students with LD experience more anxiety than their non-LD peers. Females were no more likely than males to report anxiety and levels did not differ between elementary, middle, and high school. While the authors of the meta-analysis were careful to disclose that none of the anxiety indicators in any of the 42 studies reached a clinically significant range, the higher mean anxiety scores of students with LD suggest that students with LD are more likely to experience anxiety than their non-LD peers. There was also a difference in reported anxiety levels depending on who provided the report. Self reports ($d = 0.41$) and parent reports ($d = 0.63$) were not different at a statistically significant level, but teachers consistently reported higher levels of anxiety ($d = 0.81$) among students with LD. It may be the case that anxiety depends on the setting, meaning that all assessments are valid because they reflect context-specific manifestations of anxiety (De Los Reyes & Kazdin, 2005; Grills & Ollendick, 2003). If this is the case, it may be that parents report more or less anxiety than a teacher. In addition, the context about which students think while answering their anxiety-related questions might impact their scores—are they thinking about school or home? One particular class or school in general?

Self reports of depression among students with LD have been reported as higher than those of non-LD students ($d = 0.75$; Nelson & Harwood, 2011b). Although scores do not differ significantly based on who reports depression-related symptoms (i.e., student, teacher, or parent), it is important to take all three perspectives into account, given that parent and teacher reports reflect behavioral aspects of depression while student self reports reflect the more internalized emotions associated with depression. It may be that students with LD are particularly prone to displaying behavioral symptoms of depression (e.g., moodiness and social withdrawal), making depression more noticeable to parents and teachers than are less behaviorally manifested mental health issues, such as anxiety.

Recently, Grills and Vaughn (2015) conducted a small, randomized trial investigating the preliminary efficacy and feasibility of a combined reading plus anxiety reduction intervention. A trained reading intervention teacher provided small group instruction to 35 5th-grade children randomly assigned to receive either reading plus anxiety reduction ($n = 19$) or reading-only ($n = 17$) intervention over a 5-week period. While there were no significant pre-intervention group differences for gender, reading ability, or anxiety, significant within and between group differences were found. Children in the reading plus anxiety reduction treatment demonstrated lower scores on social, generalized, and reading-related anxiety, as well as on measures of state anxiety administered prior to reading tests. Moreover, significant between group differences were found, with students in the reading plus anxiety reduction group reporting significantly reduced social and generalized anxiety at the completion of the intervention. Although these findings demonstrate the feasibility and preliminary efficacy of an integrated intervention targeting reading and anxiety, the results are preliminary and in need of larger-scale replication.

Implications for Practice

Academic interventions in reading and math are well established in schools. RTI models are now implemented across all 50 states. Almost all students with recognized LD have interaction with an academic interventionist daily. Even for students with LD who are taught exclusively in general education classes, case-workers provide academic support when needed. When we consider mental health assessment and support for students with LD, the story is quite different; they are rarely assessed for mental health needs and rarely treated in schools. School psychologists and counselors are in a particularly unique role to guide the assessment and treatment of mental health issues.

Academic progress, social emotional well-being, and mental health are related (Swanson, Harris, & Graham, 2013). Thus, considering all aspects of student success, including academic and social functioning is essential to providing the most appropriate supports. If our goal as educators and school-based mental health service providers is to close the gap between students with and without LD so that students with LD may experience a full, productive life during school and after graduation, we may need to rethink the breadth of special education service provision. While academic interventions are effective, given the pervasive existence of mental health needs among students with LD, academic interventions are simply not enough. It may be that effective academic interventions designed to combat learning difficulties, coupled with powerful mental health interventions to address social emotional difficulties, anxiety, and depression, produce a synergistic effect that tips the scales in favor of more positive outcomes for students with LD.

Take-Home Points

- The DSM-5 provides clarified and nuanced guidelines for identifying students with LD, reflecting changes in the Individuals with Disabilities Education Improvement Act of 2004.
- Using an RTI model as part of the identification process does not eliminate the requirement for a comprehensive evaluation.

- Students with LD make up 40.1% of all school-aged children identified with a disability.
- RTI models can be used to provide much-needed early intervention, particularly for ELLs who historically have had few early intervention services.
- Anxiety and depression affect most students with LD. Both academic and mental health services should be provided as part of a well-rounded intervention plan.

Resources

- Texas Center for Learning Disabilities: http://www.texasldcenter.org/
- Building RTI Capacity: http://buildingrti.utexas.org/
- National Center on Student Progress Monitoring: http://studentprogress.org/

References

American Psychiatric Association (APA). (2013). *Diagnostic and statistical manual of mental disorders* (5th ed.) (DSM-5). Washington, DC: American Psychiatric Association.

Artiles, A.J., & Ortiz, A.A. (Eds.). (2002). *English language learners with special education needs*. Washington, DC: Center for Applied Linguistics.

Barnes, A.C., & Harlacher, J.E. (2008). Clearing the confusion: Response-to-Intervention as a set of principles. *Education & Treatment of Children, 31*, 417–431.

Bowers, P.G. 2001. Exploration of the basis for rapid naming's relationship to reading. In M. Wolf (Ed.), *Dyslexia, fluency, and the brain* (pp. 41–64). Baltimore: York Press.

Bowers, P.G., & Wolf, M. (1993). Theoretical links among naming speed, precise timing mechanisms and orthographic skill in dyslexia. *Reading and Writing, 5*, 69–85.

Case, R., & Okamoto, Y. (1996). The role of central conceptual structures in the development of children's thought. *Monographs of the Society for Research in Child Development, 66* (1–2, Serial No. 246).

Catts, H.W., Compton, D., Tomblin, J.B., & Bridges, M.S. (2012). Prevalence and nature of late-emerging poor readers. *Journal of Educational Psychology, 104*(1), 166.

Crick, N.R., & Dodge, K.A. (1994). A review and reformulation of social information-processing mechanisms in children's social adjustment. *Psychological Bulletin, 115*, 74–101.

De Los Reyes, A., & Kazdin, A.E. (2005). Informant discrepancies in the assessment of childhood psychopathology: A critical review, theoretical framework, and recommendations for further study. *Psychological Bulletin, 131*(4), 483–509.

DuPaul, G.J., Gormley, M.J., & Laracy, S.D. (2013). Comorbidity of LD and ADHD: Implications of DSM-5 for assessment and treatment. *Journal of Learning Disabilities, 46*, 43–51. doi: 10.1177/0022219412464351

Elbaum, B., & Vaughn, S. (2003). Self-concept and students with learning disabilities. In H.L. Swanson, K.R. Harris, & S. Graham (Eds.), *Handbook of learning disabilities* (pp. 229–241). New York: The Guilford Press.

Estell, D.B., Jones, M.H., Pearl, R., Van Acker, R., Farmer, T.W., & Rodkin, P.C. (2008). Peer groups, popularity, and social preference trajectories of social functioning among students with and without learning disabilities. *Journal of Learning Disabilities, 41*(1), 5–14.

Fletcher, J., Steubing, K.K., Morris, R.D., & Lyon, G.R. (2013). Classification and definition of learning disabilities: A hybrid model. In H.L. Swanson, K.R. Harris, & S. Graham (Eds.), *Handbook of learning disabilities* (2nd ed., pp. 33–50). New York: The Guilford Press.

Fletcher, J. & Vaughn, S. (2009). Response to Intervention: Preventing and remediating academic difficulties. *Child Development Perspectives, 3*, 30–37.

Galway, T.M., & Metsala, J.L. (2011). Social cognition and its relation to psychosocial adjustment in children with nonverbal learning disabilities. *Journal of Learning Disabilities, 44*, 33–49.

Georgiou, G., & Parrila, R. (2013). Rapid automatized naming and reading: A review. In H.L. Swanson, K. Harris, & S. Graham (Eds.), *Handbook of learning disabilities* (2nd ed., pp. 169–185). New York: The Guilford Press.

Goswami, U. (2002). Phonology, reading development, and dyslexia: A cross-linguistic perspective. *Annals of Dyslexia, 52*, 141–163.

Grills, A.E., & Ollendick, T.H. (2003). Multiple informant agreement and the Anxiety Disorders Interview Schedule for Parents and Children. *Journal of the American Academy of Child and Adolescent Psychiatry, 42*, 30–40.

Grills, A., & Vaughn, S. (2015, manuscript in preparation). Examining the efficacy of a multi-component intervention targeting reading and anxiety.

Hallahan, D.P., Pullen, P.C., & Ward, D. (2013). A brief history of the field of learning disabilities. In H.L. Swanson, K.R. Harris, & S. Graham (Eds.), *Handbook of learning disabilities* (2nd ed., pp. 15–32). New York: The Guilford Press.

Kavale, K.A., & Forness, S.R. (1996). Social skill deficits and learning disabilities: A meta-analysis. *Journal of Learning Disabilities, 29*, 226–237.

Kirk, S. (1962). *Educating exceptional children*. Boston: Houghton Mifflin.

Kloomok, S., & Cosden, M. (1994). Self-concept in children with learning disabilities: The relationship between global self-concept, academic "discounting," nonacademic self-concept, and perceived social support. *Learning Disability Quarterly, 17*(2), 140–153.

Kovaleski, J.F., & Black, L. (2010). Multi-tier service delivery. In T.A. Glover & S. Vaughn (Eds.), *The promise of response to intervention: Evaluating current science and practice* (pp. 23–56). New York: The Guilford Press.

Lepola, J., Poskiparta, E., Laakkonen, E., & Niemi, P. (2005). Development of and relationship between phonological and motivational processes and naming speed in predicting word recognition in grade 1. *Scientific Studies of Reading, 9*(4), 367–399.

Lesaux, N.K., & Harris, J.R. (2013). Linguistically diverse students' reading difficulties: Implications for models of learning disabilities identification and effective instruction. In H.L. Swanson, K.R. Harris, & S. Graham (Eds.), *Handbook of learning disabilities* (2nd ed., pp. 69–84). New York: The Guilford Press.

Mandler, G., & Shebo, B.J. (1982). Subitizing: An analysis of its component processes. *Journal of Experimental Psychology: General, 111*, 1–22.

Margalit, M. (2010). *Lonely children and adolescents: Self-perceptions, social exclusion and hope*. New York: Springer.

McCardle, P., Mele-McCarthy, J., Cutting, L., Leos, K., & Emilio, T. (2005). Learning disabilities in English language learners: Identifying the issues. *Learning Disabilities Research and Practice, 20*(1), 1–5.

Miyake, A., Friedman, N.P., Emerson, M.J., Witzki, A.H., Howerter, A., & Wager, T.D. (2000). The unity and diversity of executive functions and their contributions to complex "frontal lobe" tasks: A latent variable analysis. *Cognitive Psychology, 41*(1), 49–100.

National Center for Learning Disabilities (Retrieved 2014). What is working memory and why does it matter? Retrieved from http://www.ncld.org/types-learning-disabilities/executive-function-disorders/what-is-working-memory-why-does-matter

Nelson, J.M., & Harwood, H. (2011a). Learning disabilities and anxiety: A meta-analysis. *Journal of Learning Disabilities, 44*, 3–17.

Nelson, J.M., & Harwood, H. (2011b). A meta-analysis of parent and teacher reports of depression among students with learning disabilities: Evidence for the importance of multi-informant assessment. *Psychology in the Schools, 48*, 371–384.

Powell, D. Stainthorp, R., Stuart, M., Garwood, H., & Quinlan, P. (2007). An experimental comparison between rival theories of rapid automatized naming performance and its relationship to reading. *Journal of Experimental Child Psychology, 98*, 46–68.

Schatschneider, C., Fletcher, J., Francis, D., Carlson, J., & Foorman, B. (2004). Kindergarten predication of reading skills: A longitudinal comparative analysis. *Journal of Educational Psychology, 96*, 265–282.

Shaywitz, S. (2004). *Overcoming dyslexia: A new and complete science-based program for reading problems at any level*. New York: Random House.

Swann, W.B. (1996). *Self-traps: The elusive quest for higher self-esteem*. New York: Freeman.

Swanson, E., & Vaughn, S. (2011). Implementing a Response to Intervention model to improve reading outcomes for all students. In S.J. Samuels & A. Farstrup (Eds.), *What research has to say about reading instruction*. International Reading Association.

Swanson, H.L., & Cochran, K. (1991). Learning disabilities, distinctive encoding and hemispheric resources. *Brain and Language, 40*, 202–230.

Swanson, H.L., Harris, K.R., & Graham, S. (Eds.). (2013). *Handbook of learning disabilities* (2nd ed.). New York: The Guilford Press.

Swanson, H.L., & Zheng, X. (2013). Memory difficulties in children and adults with learning disabilities. In H.L. Swanson, K.R. Harris, & S. Graham (Eds.), *Handbook of learning disabilities* (2nd ed., pp. 214–238). New York: The Guilford Press.

Tabassam, W., & Grainger, J. (2002). Self-concept, attributional style and self-efficacy beliefs of students with learning disabilities with and without attention deficit hyperactivity disorder. *Learning Disability Quarterly, 25*(2), 141–151.

Tannock, R. (2013). Rethinking ADHD and LD in DSM-5 Proposed Changes in Diagnostic Criteria. *Journal of Learning Disabilities, 46*(1), 5–25.

Torgesen, J.K., Wagner, R.K., & Rashotte, C.A. (1994). Longitudinal studies of phonological processing and reading. *Journal of Learning Disabilities, 27*, 276–286.

Toro, P.A., Weissberg, R.P., Guare, J., & Liebenstein, N.L. (1990). A comparison of children with and without learning disabilities on social problem-solving skills, school behavior, and family background. *Journal of Learning Disabilities, 23*, 115–120.

U.S. Department of Education. (2014). *36th Annual Report to Congress on the Implementation of the Individuals with Disabilities Education Act*. Washington, DC: Office of Special Education and Rehabilitative Services, Office of Special Education Programs.

Vellutino, F., Fletcher, J.M., Snowling, M.J., & Scanlon, D.M. (2004). Specific reading disability (dyslexia): What have we learned in the past four decades? *Journal of Child Psychology and Psychiatry, 45*, 2–40.

Wernicke, C. (1874). *Der aphasische symptomenkomplex [The symptoms of aphasia]*. Breslau, Poland: Cohn & Weigert.

Wynn, K. (1992). Children's acquisition of the number words and the counting system. *Cognitive Psychology, 24*, 220–251.

Wynn, K., Bloom, P., & Chiang, W.C. (2002). Enumeration of collective entities by 5-month-old infants. *Cognition, 83*(3), B55–B62.

5

AUTISM SPECTRUM DISORDER

Zachary Rossetti

> Children and youth with autism spectrum disorders are a particularly unique group, even when compared with other children with disabilities. The countless permutations and combinations of social interaction, language, learning, sensory, and behavior deficits and excesses found in these individuals, in combination with their wide range of abilities, developmental levels, isolated skills, and unique personalities and abilities, make autism spectrum disorders an especially baffling disability.
>
> (Simpson, 2001, p. 68)

> If I could snap my fingers and be nonautistic, I would not—because then I wouldn't be me. Autism is part of who I am.
>
> (Grandin, 1995, p. 16)

The field of autism, still in its relative infancy, has grown rapidly and changed dramatically over the last few decades. Once little known and infrequently diagnosed, autism is now a condition and topic of focus within school mental health, special education, related fields, and general society (Heward, 2013). However, despite advances there remains much that is unknown about autism, and debates about etiology and intervention persist in the field. As the excerpts above indicate, autism is inherently complex as a behaviorally based spectrum disorder and cultivates strong opinions by stakeholders. For example, while Simpson (2001) considers autism to be baffling, Grandin (1995), who is herself a woman with autism, believes it to be an important and contributing part of her identity.

Overview of Autism Spectrum Disorder

DSM-5 Diagnostic Criteria

Autism Spectrum Disorder (ASD) is a lifelong neurodevelopmental condition (or disorder), also considered a developmental disability, that is characterized by (a) persistent deficits in social communication and social interaction and (b) restricted, repetitive patterns of behavior, interests, or activities (American Psychiatric Association, 2013). The new criteria delineated in the most recent edition of the American Psychiatric Association's *Diagnostic and Statistical Manual of Mental Disorders* (DSM-5) reduced the diagnostic domains from three to two, altered the five subtypes of Pervasive Developmental Disorders (PDD) to one diagnosis of ASD, changed six out of 16 symptoms required for diagnosis to five out of seven, and broadened onset from before 3 years of age to onset in the early developmental period. The new criteria include specific examples of behaviors to characterize individual differences in presentation, severity levels based on support needs of the individual, and for the first time, a symptom based on reaction to sensory input (APA, 2013). These changes responded to the diagnostic difficulties of distinguishing between the five PDDs and of differentiating the social and communication deficits, which were separate diagnostic domains (Lord & Jones, 2012; Wing, Gould, & Gillberg, 2011). Notably, concerns persist about the consequences for individuals with profiles fitting DSM-IV but not DSM-5 criteria (Greaves-Lord et al., 2013; Wing et al., 2011).

Comorbidities

ASDs have been associated with various comorbid developmental, behavioral, and emotional disorders. As examples, language disorders, Attention-Deficit/Hyperactivity Disorder, and anxiety disorders have all been reported with high rates among people with ASD (Levy et al., 2010; Matson & Williams, 2014).

Historically, autism had been associated with comorbid rates of intellectual disability of 70–75%, with more recent figures around 40–50% (Newschaffer et al., 2007; Volkmar et al., 2014). In the most recent prevalence estimates, only 31% of children were classified within the range of intellectual disability (IQ <70), and 46% were classified with average or above average intellectual ability (Centers for Disease Control and Prevention, 2014). Calculator (2009) warned practitioners of the frequency with which individuals with ASD [and other disabilities] are misinterpreted as having a significant intellectual disability in the absence of a comprehensive and consistent means of communication.

Prevalence and Etiology

Prevalence rates of ASD have increased dramatically over the last several decades, from 1/2500 in the first epidemiologic studies during the 1960s–70s to 1/1000 in the late 1990s when the Centers for Disease Control and Prevention (CDC) established the Autism and Developmental Disabilities Monitoring (ADDM) Network to collect prevalence data for autism and other developmental disabilities in the United States (CDC, 2014; Gillberg & Wing, 1999; Newschaffer et al., 2007). Data from select ADDM sites have resulted in prevalence estimates among children aged 8 years of 6.6/1000, or about one in every 150 children, in 2002; 9.0/1000 (one in 110) in 2006; 11.3/1000 (one in 88) in 2008; and most recently, 14.7/1000 (one in 68) in 2010 (CDC, 2014). The 2010 data continued to indicate variation by sex, showing ASD is almost five times more common in boys than girls with 23.7/1000 (approximately one in 42) boys and 5.3/1000 (one in 189) girls identified with ASD (CDC, 2014). The prevalence estimates also varied by race/ethnicity with non-Hispanic white children approximately 30% more likely to be identified with ASD than non-Hispanic black children and almost 50% more likely to be identified than Hispanic children (CDC, 2014).

Awareness of these higher rates of ASD, especially in general society, fueled concerns of an autism epidemic. However, evidence supports several factors contributing to the apparent increase, such as application of broader diagnostic criteria, greater awareness of diagnostic criteria, improved diagnostic practices, and diagnostic substitution in the Individuals with Disabilities Education Act (IDEA) child count data (Fombonne, 2005; Gernsbacher, Dawson, & Goldsmith, 2005; Shattuck, 2006). Diagnostic substitution refers to statistically significant correlations between lower rates of students receiving special education services under the categories of Specific Learning Disability and Intellectual Disability corresponding to the increase in those receiving services under Autism (Shattuck, 2006).

Etiology remains a central focus within the field of autism and a source of great debate in general society. Fueled by concerns about a possible autism epidemic, fabricated data, and parental observations of developmental regression and onset of autistic symptomology, vaccines were viewed as a possible postnatal, environmental cause of ASD (Rutter, 2011). Specifically, the measles-mumps-rubella vaccine or thimerosol, the mercury-based preservative, were thought to cause ASD. To date, studies have found no increased risk or causal relationship between ASD and vaccines, nor ASD and thimerosol, despite mercury being a proven neurotoxin (Price et al., 2010; Rutter, 2011; Taylor, Swerdfeger, & Eslick, 2014).

Instead, extant research supports biological origins of ASD. Higher rates of seizure disorders and epilepsy suggest neurobiological factors play a role (Matson, Neal, Hess, Mahan, & Fodstad, 2010; Rutter, 2011). Empirical evidence also supports the importance of genetic factors with ASD. Parents who have one child with ASD have up to an 18% chance of having a second child with ASD (Ozonoff et al., 2011). Studies also show high rates of ASD in identical but not fraternal twins, particularly in males (Ozonoff et al., 2011; Rosenberg et al., 2009). Finally, ASD tends to occur more frequently in individuals with other genetic or chromosomal conditions, such as Down syndrome, Fragile X syndrome, and tuberous sclerosis (Cohen et al., 2005). It is believed that advances in identification of genetic involvement in ASD will provide the basis for biological studies seeking to detect the neural cause of ASD (Rutter, 2005).

ASD in the Early Years

Research has shown potential to identify children with ASD during the first two years of life; thus, the possibility exists for improving outcomes due to earlier intervention (Boyd, Odom, Humphreys, & Sam, 2010; National Research Council, 2001). Studies have shown early signs predictive of an ASD diagnosis (e.g., lack of joint attention skills, little eye contact, poor response to name call) to be present as early as nine months (Cangialose & Allen, 2014; Chawarska & Volkmar, 2005). Diagnosis of ASD at age 2 has been shown to have high stability at age 9 (Lord et al., 2006). However, the average age of diagnosis in the United States persists at about 4 years, and the median reported age of autism diagnosis in one study was reported at 5.7 years, suggesting that there remains a large gap during which children are without services and intervention (Shattuck et al., 2009; Zwaigenbaum et al., 2009).

Clinical diagnosis is the gold standard for ASD diagnosis, requiring careful observation through successive stages of routine developmental screening, ASD-specific screening, and comprehensive clinical evaluation. The American Academy of Pediatrics recommends surveillance for general developmental problems at the 9-, 18-, and 30-month well-child care visits and ASD-specific screening at the 18- and 24-month visits (Johnson & Myers, 2007). For broadband screening, the Infant-Toddler Checklist (ITC) (Wetherby, Brosnan-Maddox, Peace, & Newton, 2008) is a commonly used, 24-item parental questionnaire focused on social communication milestones (Boyd et al., 2010; Cangialose & Allen, 2014). Though it has been sensitive to identification of children with ASD, it is unable to distinguish between children with ASD and communication delays (Wetherby et al., 2008). For ASD-specific screening, the Modified Checklist for Autism in Toddlers (M-CHAT) (Robins, Fein, Barton, & Green, 2001) is a 23-item parent report checklist commonly used in children at least 18 months of age. Clinical diagnostic evaluation typically involves use of the Autism Diagnostic Observation Schedule (ADOS; Lord et al., 2000), a standardized assessment of communication, social interaction, play, and imagination, along with the Autism Diagnostic Interview-Revised (ADI-R; Rutter, Le Couteur, & Lord, 2003), which yields a parent/caregiver history. Ideally, such a combination of these measures is recommended.

ASD in the School Years

Students with ASD in schools should be considered in dynamic and individualized ways. The core challenge of ASD is social, but as a spectrum disorder, presentation varies across a wide range of symptoms. One student with ASD may not communicate verbally nor appear to be interested in interacting with peers, though he may desire friends. Another student with ASD may speak at length about a particular area of interest with peers, possibly without noticing others' reactions or being interested in them. Recognizing this range of differences, Kluth (2010) suggests that while individuals with ASD share commonalities, "it is critical to remember that [they] vary widely in experiences, skills, abilities, interest, characteristics, gifts, talents, and needs" (p. 2). In fact, she reminds us: "If you know one person with autism, you know ONE person with autism" (p. 2). In practice, this means that awareness of an ASD diagnosis is just the starting point towards the assessment-based development of individualized education programs.

School Experiences and Risk Factors

While individualization is critical, the school mental health context for students with ASD also consists of patterns of special education service delivery, social experiences, and school completion. Despite overall increased rates of inclusive education (i.e., participation and special education service delivery in general education classrooms), only 39% of students receiving special education and related services under the IDEA category of autism spent more than 80% of the day in the general education classroom compared to 61% of students with any disability (U.S. Department of Education, 2013). One third (33.7%) of students with autism spent less than 40% of the day in the general education classroom (U.S. Department of Education, 2013). These figures could be interpreted to mean that students with ASD have such intensive needs that the general education classroom is not their least restrictive environment. However, analysis of placement of students with ASD by state revealed a wide range of percentages of students in inclusive, mainstream, self-contained, and separate settings, suggesting that factors external to student characteristics affect placement decisions (Kurth, 2014). Placement and program decisions must be based on comprehensive educational evaluations detailing student needs and strengths.

Though the core challenge in ASD is social, many students with ASD have shown that they desire friendships despite these difficulties (Bauminger & Kasari, 2000; Calder, Hill, & Pellicano, 2012). However, social outcomes for students with ASD remain low compared to peers with other disabilities (Cadwallader & Wagner, 2002; Wagner, Cadwallader, & Marder, 2003). Students with ASD had smaller and lower quality social networks, less reciprocal and lower quality friendships, and greater social isolation than their peers without disabilities (Kasari, Locke, Gulsrud, & Rotheram-Fuller, 2011; Locke, Ishijima, Kasari, & London, 2010). One critical factor is the frequent assignment of special education paraprofessionals to students with ASD as paraprofessional proximity hinders social opportunities between students with and without ASD (Broer, Doyle, & Giangreco, 2005; Giangreco, Suter, & Doyle, 2010).

Recent data show that 87.5% of students with ASD graduated high school, which is on par with other students who received special education services (Institute of Education Sciences, 2009). Despite secondary school completion, adult outcomes have historically been interpreted as poor for individuals with ASD (Henninger & Taylor, 2012). Adults with ASD have been reported to experience low rates of competitive employment and postsecondary education, and the lowest rates of independent living among those with disabilities who received special education services (Anderson, Shattuck, Cooper, Roux, & Wagner, 2014). One factor is the transition plan and process, during which students with ASD were less likely to take leadership roles and to have transition goals related to competitive employment, postsecondary education, and independent living compared to peers with other disabilities (Shogren & Plotner, 2012).

Individualized Instruction and Evidence-based Intervention

Reflective of the core challenge of ASD, the first consideration in developing individualized instruction and intervention approaches should be social. All students with ASD should have social goals in their IEPs and/or a focus on social skills and interactions at school. Core interventions include social skills instruction, peer-mediated approaches, facilitation of social opportunities, and communication supports. Social skills instruction may take a variety of forms but should be systematic, explicit, and visual (Bellini, 2008; Simpson, Ganz, & Mason, 2012). Evidence-based practices include video modeling, social skills groups, Social Stories™, script-based interventions, and peer-mediated approaches (Bellini & Akullian, 2007; Reichow & Volkmar, 2009; Wang & Spillane, 2009). Peer-mediated approaches, which include peer tutoring, peer buddies, and other forms of peer support, increase access to the general education curriculum, decrease reliance on paraprofessional support, and facilitate social interactions with peers (Carter, Sisco, Chung, & Stanton-Chapman, 2010).

Facilitation of social opportunities consists of intentional, individualized strategies to support individuals with ASD and classmates to interact consistently over time. Facilitation strategies include, but are not limited to, pairing students based on shared interests, connecting students through shared projects, helping students with ASD negotiate social situations, and teaching peers how best to interact with classmates with ASD (Bauminger & Shulman, 2003; Hollingsworth & Buysse, 2009; Rossetti & Goessling, 2010). Facilitation by educators and parents has contributed to friendships between some students with ASD and peers without disabilities (Bauminger & Shulman, 2003; Rossetti, 2012).

Communication supports are vital for students with ASD because of the impact of communication on social interaction, behavioral presentation, and academic performance. As with social skills, students with ASD should have communication goals on their IEPs with intervention provided by a speech-language pathologist. Communication by individuals with ASD may comprise speech;

unaided augmentative and alternative communication (AAC) modes, such as manual signing and physical gestures; and aided AAC, including picture symbols, communication books, and voice output communication aids (Mirenda, 2003). Intervention ranges from social pragmatics groups (for those who speak fluently) to individual speech therapy (for those who speak with difficulty) to AAC use (for those who do not speak). Evidence exists supporting the effectiveness of the Picture Exchange Communication System and voice output communication aids, as well as, to a lesser degree, communication boards, gestures, and sign language (Ganz et al., 2012). The use of AAC does not decrease speech production and may support increased speech by allowing students to focus on communication and language skills rather than struggling with speech production (Millar, Light, & Schlosser, 2006).

Educational programs for students with ASD should consist of structured educational and behavioral interventions (National Research Council, 2001). Structured teaching responds directly to a pattern in individuals with ASD of shared strengths and challenges that the originators of the structured teaching approach call the *Culture of Autism* (Mesibov et al., 2005). The Culture of Autism includes: (a) relative strength in processing visual information; (b) increased attention to details but difficulties deriving meaning from them; (c) variability in attention; (d) communication difficulties, especially with initiating and using language socially; (e) difficulty with conceptual understanding of time; (f) tendency to become attached to routines and the settings in which they were established, resulting in difficulties with generalization; (g) strong interests and impulses to engage in favored activities, as well as difficulty disengaging from them; and (h) sensory preferences and dislikes. To address these, structured teaching consists of four primary components: (a) structuring the environment and activities in ways that are understandable to the student with ASD, (b) using students' strengths in visual skills (i.e., use of activity schedules and visual cues) to supplement relatively weaker skills, (c) using students' interests to engage them in learning, and (d) supporting self-initiated use of meaningful communication (Mesibov & Shea, 2010). Research supports the efficacy of TEACCH (Treatment and Education of Autistic and related Communication-handicapped CHildren) and the Early Start Denver Model (Dawson et al., 2010; Mesibov & Shea, 2010).

Behavioral interventions guided by the principles and methods of Applied Behavior Analysis (ABA) can be used effectively to increase expected behaviors, decrease unexpected behaviors, teach new skills, and generalize behaviors and skills in new environments or contexts (Myers & Johnson, 2007). ABA-based interventions utilize empirically supported practices, but are often administered in clinical or one-on-one settings; thus, emphasis on generalization is critical (Alberto & Troutman, 2013). Early Intensive Behavioral Intervention (EIBI) is one of the most commonly used and empirically supported ABA-based interventions (Reichow, 2012). Despite claims that certain comprehensive treatment models, such as EIBI, are more empirically supported and effective than others, there is growing consensus from researchers, practitioners, and families that supports a combination of approaches based on the unique needs of the child (Callahan, Shukla-Mehta, Magee, & Wie, 2010; Odom, Hume, Boyd, & Stabel, 2012). This individualized approach fits well within special education policy and practice.

Positive behavior support (PBS) is an applied science with foundations in ABA, the principles of normalization and inclusion, and person-centered values that emphasizes prevention of unexpected or maladaptive behaviors through individualization of behavioral supports and strategies (Carr et al., 2002). PBS-based interventions, such as Functional Behavior Assessment (FBA) which aims to identify the function of a student's behavior, are established evidence-based practices (Odom, Collet-Klingenberg, Rogers, & Hatton, 2010). FBAs are not interventions per se, but have been mandated by the Individuals with Disabilities Education Act since 1997 to guide the development of interventions and behavioral intervention plans aimed at the reduction of challenging behaviors (Heward, 2013). Administering a formal, comprehensive FBA is highly recommended prior to making any decisions relative to a student's behaviors.

Students with ASD often receive intervention or consultation from occupational therapists related to sensory modulation symptoms. As many as 45 to 95% of individuals with ASD have shown sensory processing difficulties or sensory-related behaviors (Ben-Sasson et al., 2009). Sensory integration therapy (SIT), an assessment-based program of sensory activities (e.g., wearing a weighted vest, being brushed, swinging, being squeezed or receiving pressure) designed to improve the nervous system's ability to process sensory stimuli, is among the most commonly administered interventions for students with ASD (Lang et al., 2012). Despite its widespread use, the research base supporting the effectiveness of SIT as an evidence-based practice is not yet established (Lang et al., 2012). Research on SIT and other sensory interventions is ongoing. Nonetheless, due to the common experience of sensory modulation symptoms, occupational therapists should be included on the school team for students with ASD.

Take-Home Points

- Though the field of autism is still in its relative infancy, empirical evidence supports a growing list of comprehensive treatment models and focused interventions.
- All students with ASD are different; thus, individualization of educational programming, mental health supports, and special education and related services is critical.
- Maintaining high expectations (e.g., presuming competence) for students with ASD is critical because we cannot know what someone is thinking based on his or her behaviors.
- Though ASD is a neurological condition, structured educational and behavioral interventions have been shown to be effective for students with ASD.

- Visual supports (e.g., schedules, behavior charts, physical or visual prompts) help students with ASD understand expectations and routines in the environment.
- As students with ASD age, the special education transition process needs to be improved in order to achieve better adult outcomes.

Resources

- The Infant-Toddler Checklist (ITC): http://firstwords.fsu.edu/index.php/early-identification-of-communication-delays/26-csbschecklist
- The Modified Checklist for Autism in Toddlers (M-CHAT): http://www.mchatscreen.com/Official_M-CHAT_Website.html
- For a complete listing of evidence-based practices for students with ASD, refer to:
  - The National Autism Center's *Evidence-Based Practice and Autism in the Schools*: http://www.nationalautismcenter.org/pdf/NAC%20Ed%20Manual_FINAL.pdf
  - The National Professional Development Center on Autism Spectrum Disorders' *Evidence-Based Practices for Children, Youth, and Young Adults with Autism Spectrum* Disorder: http://autismpdc.fpg.unc.edu/sites/autismpdc.fpg.unc.edu/files/2014-EBP-Report.pdf
- For professional development in established and emerging interventions and approaches, refer to Autism Internet Modules: http://www.autisminternet-modules.org

References

Alberto, P.A., & Troutman, A.C. (2013). *Applied behavior analysis for teachers* (9th ed.). Boston, MA: Pearson.

American Psychiatric Association (APA). (2013). *Diagnostic and statistical manual of mental disorders* (5th ed.) (DSM-5). Washington, DC: American Psychiatric Association.

Anderson, K.A., Shattuck, P.T., Cooper, B.P., Roux, A.M., & Wagner, M. (2014). Prevalence and correlates of postsecondary residential status among young adults with an autism spectrum disorder. *Autism, 18*, 562–570. doi: 10.1177/1362361313481860

Bauminger, N., & Kasari, C. (2000) Loneliness and friendship in high-functioning children with autism. *Child Development, 71*, 447–456.

Bauminger, N., & Shulman, C. (2003). The development and maintenance of friendship in high-functioning children with autism: Maternal perceptions. *Autism, 7*, 81–97.

Bellini, S. (2008). *Building social relationships: A systematic approach to teaching social interaction skills to children and adolescents with autism spectrum disorders and other social difficulties*. Shawnee Mission, KS: Autism Asperger Publishing Co.

Bellini, S., & Akullian, J. (2007). A meta-analysis of video modeling and video self-modeling interventions for children and adolescents with autism spectrum disorders. *Exceptional Children, 73*, 261–284.

Ben-Sasson, A., Hen, L., Fluss, R., Cermak, S.A., Engel-Yeger, B., & Gal, E. (2009). A meta-analysis of sensory modulation symptoms in individuals with autism spectrum disorders. *Journal of Autism and Developmental Disorders, 39*, 1–11. doi: 10.1007/s10803–008–0593–3

Boyd, B.A., Odom, S.L., Humphreys, B.P., & Sam, A.M. (2010). Infants and toddlers with autism spectrum disorder: Early identification and early intervention. *Journal of Early Intervention, 32*, 75–98.

Broer, S.M., Doyle, M.B., & Giangreco, M.F. (2005). Perspectives of students with intellectual disabilities about their experiences with paraprofessional support. *Exceptional Children, 71*(4), 415–430.

Cadwallader, T.W., & Wagner, M. (2002). Students' interactions with friends. In M. Wagner, T. Cadwallader, C. Marder, L. Newman, N. Garza, & J. Blackorby (Eds.), *The other 80% of their time: The experiences of elementary and middle school students with disabilities in their non-school hours* (pp. 4.1–4.7). Menlo Park, CA: SRI International.

Calculator, S.N. (2009). Augmentative and alternative communication (AAC) and inclusive education for students with the most severe disabilities. *International Journal of Inclusive Education, 13*, 93–113.

Calder, L., Hill, V., & Pellicano, E. (2012). "Sometimes I want to play by myself": Understanding what friendship means to children with autism in mainstream primary schools. *Autism, (17)*, 296–316. doi: 10.1177/1362361312467866

Callahan, K., Shukla-Mehta, S., Magee, S., & Wie, M. (2010). ABA versus TEACCH: The case for defining and validating comprehensive treatment models in autism. *Journal of Autism and Developmental Disorders, 40*, 74–88. doi: 10.1007/s10803–009–0834–0

Cangialose, A., & Allen, P.J. (2014). Screening for autism spectrum disorders in infants before 18 months of age. *Pediatric Nursing, 40*, 33–37.

Carr, E.G., Dunlap, G., Horner, R.H., Koegel, R.L., Turnbull, A.P., Sailor, W., . . . Fox, L. (2002). Positive behavior support: Evolution of an applied science. *Journal of Positive Behavior Interventions, 4*, 4–16.

Carter, E.W., Sisco, L.G., Chung, Y., & Stanton-Chapman, T.L. (2010). Peer interactions of students with intellectual disabilities and/or autism: A map of the intervention literature. *Research and Practice for Persons with Severe Disabilities, 35*, 63–79.

Centers for Disease Control and Prevention (CDC). (2014). Prevalence of autism spectrum disorder among children aged 8 years: Autism and developmental disabilities monitoring network, 11 sites, United States, 2010. *MMWR Surveillance Summaries, 63*(2), 1–22.

Chawarska, K., & Volkmar, F.R. (2005). Autism in infancy and early childhood. In F.R. Volkmar, R. Paul, A. Klin, & D. Cohen (Eds.), *Handbook of autism and pervasive developmental disorders, volume one: Diagnosis, development, neurobiology, and behavior* (3rd ed., pp. 223–246). Hoboken, NJ: Wiley.

Cohen, D., Pichard, N., Tordjman, S., Baumann, C., Burglen, L., Excoffier, E., . . . Heron, D. (2005). Specific genetic disorders and autism: Clinical contribution towards their identification. *Journal of Autism and Developmental Disorders, 35*, 103–116. doi: 0162–3257/05/0200–0103/0

Dawson, G., Rogers, S., Munson, J., Smith, M., Winter, J., Greenson, J., . . . Varley, J. (2010). Randomized, controlled trial of an intervention for toddlers with autism: The Early Start Denver Model. *Pediatrics, 125*, e17–e23. doi: 10.1542/peds.2009–0958

Fombonne, E. (2005). Epidemiological studies of pervasive developmental disorders. In F.R. Volkmar, R. Paul, A. Klin, & D. Cohen (Eds.), *Handbook of autism and pervasive developmental disorders, volume one: Diagnosis, development, neurobiology, and behavior* (3rd ed., pp. 42–69). Hoboken, NJ: Wiley.

Ganz, J.B., Earles-Vollrath, T.L., Heath, A.K., Parker, R.I., Rispoli, M.J., & Duran, J.B. (2012). A meta-analysis of single case research studies on aided augmentative and alternative communication systems with individuals with autism spectrum disorders. *Journal of Autism and Developmental Disorders, 42*, 60–74. doi: 10.1007/s10803–011–1212–2

Gernsbacher, M.A., Dawson, M., & Goldsmith, H.H. (2005). Three reasons not to believe in an autism epidemic. *Current Directions in Psychological Science, 14*, 55–58.

Giangreco, M.F., Suter, J.C., & Doyle, M.B. (2010). Paraprofessionals in inclusive schools: A review of recent research. *Journal of Educational and Psychological Consultation, 20*, 41–57.

Gillberg, C., & Wing, L. (1999). Autism: Not an extremely rare disorder. *Acta Psychiatrica Scandinavica, 99*, 399–406.

Grandin, T. (1995). *Thinking in pictures and other reports from my life with autism*. New York, NY: Vintage Books.

Greaves-Lord, K., Eussen, M.L.J.M., Verhulst, F.C., Minderaa, R.B., Mandy, W., Hudziak, J.J., . . . Hartman, C.A. (2013). Empirically based phenotypic profiles of children with pervasive developmental disorders: Interpretation in the light of the DSM-5. *Journal of Autism and other Developmental Disorders, 43*, 1784–1797. doi: 10.1007/s10803–012–1724–4

Henninger, N.A., & Taylor, J.L. (2012). Outcomes in adults with autism spectrum disorders: A historical perspective. *Autism, 17*, 103–116. doi: 10.1177/1362361312441266

Heward, W.L. (2013). *Exceptional children: An introduction to special education* (10th ed.). Upper Saddle River, NJ: Merrill.

Hollingsworth, H.L., & Buysse, V. (2009). Establishing friendships in early childhood inclusive settings. *Journal of Early Intervention, 31*, 287–307.

Institute of Education Sciences (IES) National Center for Special Education Research. (2009). National Longitudinal Transition Study 2 [Data file]. Retrieved from http://www.nlts2.org/data_tables/tables/14/np5S1a_A2efrm.html

Johnson, C.P., & Myers, S.M. (2007). Identification and evaluation of children with autism spectrum disorders. *Pediatrics, 120*, 1183–1215. doi: 10.1542/peds.2007–2361

Kasari, C., Locke, J., Gulsrud, A., & Rotheram-Fuller, E. (2011). Social networks and friendships at school: Comparing children with and without ASD. *Journal of Autism and Developmental Disorders, 41*, 533–544. doi: 10.1007/s10803–010–1076-x

Kluth, P. (2010). *"You're going to love this kid!": Teaching students with autism in the inclusive classroom* (2nd ed.). Baltimore: Paul H. Brookes.

Kurth, J.A. (2014). Educational placement of students with autism: The impact of state of residence. *Focus on Autism and Other Developmental Disabilities*. doi: 10.1177/1088357614547891.

Lang, R., O'Reilly, M., Healy, O., Rispoli, M., Lydon, H., Streusand, W., . . . Giesbers, S. (2012). Sensory integration therapy for autism spectrum disorders: A systematic review. *Research in Autism Spectrum Disorders, 6*, 1004–1018. doi: 10.1016/j.rasd.2012.01.006

Levy, S.E., Giarelli, E., Lee, L., Schieve, L., Kirby, R.S., Cunniff, C., . . . Rice, C.E. (2010). Autism spectrum disorder and co-occurring developmental, psychiatric, and medical conditions among children in multiple populations of the United States. *Journal of Developmental & Behavioral Pediatrics, 31*, 267–275. doi: 10.1097/DBP.0b013e3181d5d03b

Locke, J., Ishijima, E.H., Kasari, C., & London, N. (2010). Loneliness, friendship quality and social networks of adolescents with high-functioning autism in an inclusive school setting. *Journal of Research in Special Education Needs, 10*, 74–81.

Lord, C., & Jones, R.M. (2012). Annual research review: Re-thinking the classification of autism spectrum disorders. *The Journal of Child Psychology and Psychiatry, 53*, 490–509. doi: 10.1111/j.1469–7610.2012.02547.x

Lord, C., Risi, S., DiLavore, P.S., Shulman, C., Thurm, A., & Pickles, A. (2006). Autism from 2 to 9 years of age. *Archives of General Psychiatry, 6*, 694–701.

Lord, C., Risi, S., Lambrecht, L., Cook, E.H., Leventhal, B.L., DiLavore, P.C., Pickles, A., & Rutter, M. (2000). The autism diagnostic observation schedule-generic: A standard measure of social and communication deficits associated with the spectrum of autism. *Journal of Autism and Developmental Disorders, 30*, 205–223.

Matson, J.L., Neal, D., Hess, J.A., Mahan, S., & Fodstad, J.C. (2010). The effect of seizure disorder on symptom presentation in atypically developing children and children with autism spectrum disorders based on the BDI-2. *Developmental Neurorehabilitation, 13*, 310–314. doi: 10.3109/17518421003782192

Matson, J.L., & Williams, L.W. (2014). Depression and mood disorders among persons with autism spectrum disorders. *Research in Developmental Disabilities, 35*, 2003–2007. doi: 10.1016/j.ridd.2014.04.020

Mesibov, G.B., & Shea, V. (2010). The TEACCH program in the era of evidence-based practice. *Journal of Autism and Developmental Disorders, 40*, 570–579. doi: 10.1007/s10803–009–0901–6

Mesibov, G.B., Shea, V., & Schopler, E. (with Adams, L., Burgess, S., Chapman, S.M., Merkler, E., Mosconi, M., Tanner, C., & Van Bourgondien, M.E.). (2005). *The TEACCH approach to autism spectrum disorders*. New York: Springer.

Millar, D.C., Light, J.C., & Schlosser, R.W. (2006). The impact of augmentative and alternative communication intervention on the speech production of individuals with developmental disabilities: A research review. *Journal of Speech, Language, and Hearing Research, 49*, 248–264.

Mirenda, P. (2003). Toward functional augmentative and alternative communication for students with autism: Manual signs, graphic symbols, and voice output communication aids. *Language, Speech, and Hearing Services in Schools, 34*, 203–216.

Myers, S.M., & Johnson, C.P. (2007). Management of children with autism spectrum disorders. *Pediatrics, 120*, 1162–1182. doi: 10.1542/peds.2007–2362

National Research Council. (2001). *Educating children with autism*. Washington, DC: National Academy Press.

Newschaffer, C.J., Croen, L.A., Daniels, J., Giarelli, E., Grether, J.K., Levy, S.E., . . . Windham, G.C. (2007). The epidemiology of autism spectrum disorders. *Annual Review of Public Health, 28*, 235–258. doi: 10.1146/annurev.publhealth.28.021406.144007

Odom, S.L., Collet-Klingenberg, L., Rogers, S.J., & Hatton, D.D. (2010). Evidence-based practices in interventions for children and youth with autism spectrum disorders. *Preventing School Failure, 54*, 275–282. doi: 10.1080/10459881003785506

Odom, S., Hume, K., Boyd, B., & Stabel, A. (2012). Moving beyond the intensive behavior treatment versus eclectic dichotomy: Evidence-based and individualized programs for learners with ASD. *Behavior Modification, 36*, 270–297. doi: 10.1177/0145445512444595

Ozonoff, S., Young, G.S., Carter, A., Messinger, D., Yirmiya, N., Zwaigenbaum, L., . . . Stone, W.L. (2011). Recurrence risk for autism spectrum disorders: A baby siblings research consortium study. *Pediatrics, 128*, e488–e495. doi: 10.1542/peds.2010-2825

Price, C.S., Thompson, W.W., Goodson, B., Weintraub, E.S., Croen, L.A., Hinrichsen, V.L., . . . DeStefano, F. (2010). Prenatal and infant exposure to thimerosol from vaccines and immunoglobulins and risk of autism. *Pediatrics, 126*, 656–664.

Reichow, B. (2012). Overview of meta-analyses on Early Intensive Behavioral Intervention for young children with autism spectrum disorders. *Journal of Autism and Developmental Disorders, 42*, 512–520. doi: 10.1007/s10803-011-1218-9

Reichow, B., & Volkmar, F.R. (2009). Social skills interventions for individuals with autism: Evaluation for evidence-based practices within a best evidence synthesis framework. *Journal of Autism and Developmental Disorders, 40*, 149–166. doi: 10.1007/s10803-009-0842-0

Robins, D.L., Fein, D., Barton, M.L., & Green, J.A. (2001). The Modified Checklist for Autism in Toddlers: An initial study investigating the early detection of autism and pervasive developmental disorders. *Journal of Autism and Developmental Disorders, 31*, 131–144. doi: 0162-3257/01/0400-0131

Rosenberg, R.E., Law, J.K., Yenokyan, G., McGready, J., Kaufmann, W.E., & Law, P.A. (2009). Characteristics and concordance of autism spectrum disorders among 277 twin pairs. *Archives of Pediatrics & Adolescent Medicine, 163*, 907–914. doi: 10.1001/archpediatrics.2009.98

Rossetti, Z. (2012). Helping or hindering: The role of secondary educators in facilitating friendship opportunities among students with and without autism or developmental disability. *International Journal of Inclusive Education, 16*, 1259–1272. doi: 10.1080/13603116.2011.557448

Rossetti, Z., & Goessling, D. (2010). The role of paraeducators in facilitating friendships between high school students with and without autism or other developmental disabilities. *TEACHING Exceptional Children, 42*(6), 64–70.

Rutter, M. (2005). Genetic influences and autism. In F.R. Volkmar, R. Paul, A. Klin, & D. Cohen (Eds.), *Handbook of autism and pervasive developmental disorders, volume one: Diagnosis, development, neurobiology, and behavior* (3rd ed., pp. 425–452). Hoboken, NJ: Wiley.

Rutter, M.L. (2011). Progress in understanding autism: 2007–2010. *Journal of Autism and Developmental Disorders, 41*, 395–404. doi: 10.1007/s10803-011-1184-2

Rutter, M., Le Couteur, A., & Lord, C. (2003). *Autism diagnostic interview-revised—WPS* (WPS ed.). Los Angeles: Western Psychological Services.

Shattuck, P.T. (2006). The contribution of diagnostic substitution to the growing administrative prevalence of autism in US special education. *Pediatrics, 117*, 1028–1037. doi: 10.1542/peds.2005-1516

Shattuck, P.T., Durkin, M., Maenner, M., Newschaffer, C., Mandell, D.S., Wiggins, L., . . . Cuniff, C. (2009). Timing of identification among children with an autism spectrum disorder: Findings from a population-based surveillance study. *Journal of the American Academy of Child & Adolescent Psychiatry, 48*, 474–483. doi: 10.1097/CHI.0b013e31819b3848

Shogren, K.A., & Plotner, A.J. (2012). Transition planning for students with intellectual disability, autism, or other disabilities: Data from the National Longitudinal Transition Study-2. *Intellectual and Developmental Disabilities, 50*, 16–30. doi: 10.1352/1934-9556-50.1.16

Simpson, R.L. (2001). ABA and students with autism spectrum disorders: Issues and considerations for effective practice. *Focus on Autism and Other Developmental Disabilities, 16*, 68–71.

Simpson, R.L., Ganz, J.B., & Mason, R. (2012). Social skills interventions and programming for learners with autism spectrum disorders. In D. Zager, M.L. Wehmeyer, & R.L. Simpson (Eds.), *Educating students with autism spectrum disorders: Research-based principles and practices* (pp. 207–226). New York, NY: Routledge.

Taylor, L.E., Swerdfeger, A.L., & Eslick, G.D. (2014). Vaccines are not associated with autism: An evidence-based meta-analysis of case control and cohort studies. *Vaccine, 32*, 3623–3629. doi: 10.1016/j.vaccine.2014.04.085

U.S. Department of Education. (2013). *35th Annual Report to Congress on the Implementation of the Individuals with Disabilities Education Act*. Washington, DC: Office of Special Education and Rehabilitative Services, Office of Special Education Programs.

Volkmar, F., Siegel, M., Woodbury-Smith, M., King, B., McCracken, J., State, M., & the American Academy of Child and Adolescent Psychiatry (AACAP) Committee on Quality Issues (CQI). (2014). Practice parameter for the assessment and treatment of children and adolescents with autism spectrum disorder. *Journal of the American Academy of Child & Adolescent Psychiatry, 53*, 237–257. doi: 10.1016/j.jaac.2013.10.013

Wagner, M., Cadwallader, T.W., & Marder, C. (2003). *Life outside the classroom for youth with disabilities: A report from the National Longitudinal Study-2 (NLTS2).* Menlo Park, CA: SRI International.

Wang, P., & Spillane, A. (2009). Evidence-based social skills interventions for children with autism: A meta-analysis. *Education and Training in Developmental Disabilities, 44*, 318–342.

Wetherby, A.M., Brosnan-Maddox, S., Peace, V., & Newton, L. (2008). Validation of the Infant-Toddler Checklist as a broadband screener for autism spectrum disorders from 9 to 24 months of age. *Autism, 12*, 487–511. doi: 10.1177/1362361308094501

Wing, L., Gould, J., & Gillberg, C. (2011). Autism spectrum disorders in the DSM-V: Better or worse than the DSM-IV? *Research in Developmental Disabilities, 32*, 768–773. doi: 10.1016/j.ridd.2010.11.003

Zwaigenbaum, L., Bryson, S., Lord, C., Rogers, S., Carter, A., Carver, L., . . . Yirmiya, N. (2009). Clinical assessment and management of toddlers with suspected autism spectrum disorder: Insights from studies of high-risk infants. *Pediatrics, 123*, 1383–1391. doi: 10.1542/peds.2008-1606

6

SUBSTANCE USE

Heidemarie Blumenthal, Lindsay S. Ham, Renee M. Cloutier, and Alexander J. Melkonian

Adolescent substance use is linked to an array of neurological (Squeglia, Jacobus, & Tapert, 2009), mental health (e.g., anxiety; Saraceno, Munafò, Heron, Craddock, & van den Bree, 2009), behavioral (e.g., sexual risk-taking; Miller, Levy, Spicer, & Taylor, 2006), and academic (Townsend, Flisher, & King, 2007) problems. Nonetheless, experimentation with substance use, and the initiation of alcohol, cigarette, and marijuana use in particular, is common among youth (Kann et al., 2014). Schools represent an important context in which substance use could be prevented, reduced, or even promoted, posing unique opportunities for intervention. Researchers have noted the limitations of traditional clinic-based service delivery methods in reaching a large number of adolescents that may be addressed via school-based assessments and interventions (see Wagner, Tubman, & Gil, 2004). The present chapter focuses on critical issues surrounding substance use (e.g., prevalence, etiology, correlates) and evidence-based practices for assessment and intervention in school settings.

Scope of the Problem

Prevalence

Findings from the 2013 Centers for Disease Control and Prevention (CDC)-sponsored Youth Risk Behavior Surveillance Survey (YRBSS) indicated that among U.S. 12th graders, 75.6% had tried alcohol, 48.1% cigarettes, 48.6% marijuana, and 21.3% prescription drugs (for nonmedical purposes) in their lifetime, far exceeding rates of other illicit substances, including heroin (2.2%), cocaine (5.5%), and ecstasy (6.6%). Although reported use of alcohol, cigarettes, and marijuana among youth has significantly declined over the past two decades (Kann et al., 2014), adolescent substance use remains a problem. Preliminary data regarding the use of alternative nicotine uptake mechanisms (e.g., e-cigarettes, hookah) show a sharp increase, off-setting noted declines in adolescent use of more traditional tobacco products (National Youth Tobacco Survey; CDC, 2014). In addition, recent data suggest that marijuana use rates may be stabilizing (Kann et al., 2014), and targeted assessment of prescription drug misuse has only recently been introduced.

There is considerable variation in subsequent substance use patterns and trajectories. Although most adolescents do not engage in problematic use (e.g., Brown et al., 2008), a significant subset of adolescents do progress to risk-related consumption. For instance, 5.6% of U.S. high school students report frequent cigarette use (i.e. ≥ 20 of the past 30 days) and 20.8% report past-30-day binge drinking (i.e. ≥5 drinks within ~2 hours; Kann et al., 2014). Further, the Munich Early Developmental Stages of Psychopathology study found that 7.4% of youth ages 14–17 years met criteria for a DSM-IV lifetime alcohol use disorder, 12.5% for lifetime nicotine dependence, and 2.6% lifetime cannabis use disorder (Wittchen et al., 2007). As adolescents progress more rapidly from initial use to substance-related problems as compared to adults (Deas, Riggs, Langenbucher, Goldman, & Brown, 2000), and risk-related use among youth is positively correlated with problematic use in adulthood (Brown et al., 2008), preventing or delaying initiation during adolescence could prevent problems from developing or reduce their subsequent severity.

Learning and Academic Outcomes

The rapid neurological and somatic development that characterizes adolescence sets the stage for distinct acute and long-term effects of substance use as compared to adults (e.g., attenuated motor impairment, enhanced neurological damage; Windle et al., 2008). Academic achievement not only is impacted by the deleterious effects of acute intoxication and immediate after-effects (Jeynes, 2002), but substance use also consistently evidences positive relations with long-term academic difficulties (Bryant, Schulenberg, O'Malley, Bachman, & Johnston, 2003) and school dropout (Townsend et al., 2007). Importantly, this literature indicates a complex relation; some work highlights substance use as a predictor of school truancy and drop out (e.g., Roebuck, French, & Dennis, 2004), other work finds that academic problems and/or drop out predict increased substance use (e.g., Bryant et al., 2003), and others emphasize the role of shared-factors (e.g., non-conformity broadly; Townsend et al., 2007) or indirect effects linking use and academic achievement (e.g., sleep; James, Kristjánsson, & Sigfúsdóttir, 2011). Although support for the bi-directional nature of academic difficulties and substance use has been found for alcohol, cigarette, and marijuana independently, the majority of this literature has used composite variables (e.g., frequency of *any* substance use), a wide range of use indices (e.g., lifetime use, frequent use), and varying operational definitions (e.g., 'recent' use as past 7-day, 30-day; Townsend et al., 2007). Further, limited work has examined key developmental (parental support), contextually relevant (e.g., teacher support), or individual difference variables (e.g., internalization of academic goals) as potential moderators of the substance use-academic functioning association. Given theoretical and empirical support for expecting a link between adolescent substance use and academic functioning (Townsend et al., 2007), data regarding the direct, indirect, and multivariate relations relevant to intervention efforts clearly are needed.

Developmental Etiology of Adolescent Substance Use

An extensive body of work demonstrates the equifinality of adolescent substance use problems. Several excellent reviews (e.g., Brown et al., 2008; Dawes et al., 2000; Saraceno, et al., 2009) examine developmentally salient risk and protective factors. In addition to genetic and neurological correlates, cognitive aspects (e.g., perceived risk), personality factors (e.g., sensation seeking), as well as familial and peer use and attitudes have received the greatest attention, and support, in this literature. For example, the National Institutes of Health-sponsored Monitoring the Future (MTF) study consistently indicates negative relations among adolescent-reported disapproval/perceived risk and substance use among youth in the U.S. (Johnston, O'Malley, Miech, Bachman, & Schulenberg 2015). Indeed, alongside the recent stabilization in adolescent marijuana use reported by the CDC (Kann et al., 2014), the MTF study found significant declines in perceived risk and disapproval of marijuana use among 8th–12th grade youth. Further, particular substance use expectancies and motives may set the stage for the development of problematic behaviors. Enhancement and social motives for alcohol use are the most commonly endorsed among youth, whereas coping motives are most strongly associated with current and subsequent problems. Conformity motives also are related to problematic use, but may represent the primary motive among early users who have yet to internalize alternative patterns (Cooper, 1994). As both cognitive development (e.g., complexity of the coping repertoire) and experience with substances progress across adolescence, this period marks a sensitive window for the learning and maintenance of substance use patterns.

Developmentally relevant personality factors (e.g., sensation seeking, anxiety) consistently evidence positive links with concurrent and prospective substance use (Sargent, Tanski, Stoolmiller, & Hanewinkel, 2010) and disorder (Sher, Bartholow, & Wood, 2000). In a sample of over 5,500 youth, Sargent and colleagues (2010) found that baseline sensation seeking (at ages 10–14) prospectively predicted both onset of binge drinking (77% were "high" sensation seekers) and established smoking (>100 cigarettes in lifetime; 92% were "high" sensation seekers). Factors such as anxiety sensitivity (i.e. fear of anxiety-relevant sensations) and relevant constellations of anxiety symptoms (e.g., social anxiety) also demonstrate unique predictive validity in terms risk-related motives and diagnostic status (e.g., Blumenthal, Leen-Feldner, Badour, Babson, 2011).

Finally, external agents in the microsystem (e.g., family, peers), evidence multifaceted influences on adolescent substance use. Parent and sibling use are positively associated with adolescent substance use and coping-related motives (Windle, 2000). In addition to shared genetic and related environmental features (e.g., gene-environment correlations), these links may be derived from direct modeling, indirect effects via family functioning (e.g., increased conflict; decreased communication), as well as transmission of substance-positive attitudes. As adolescence progresses, youth seek greater autonomy from the family, and the role of peers increases in import and impact. Consistent with this process, actual and *perceived* peer use uniquely contribute to adolescent substance use outcomes (Sitnick, Shaw, & Hyde, 2014). Building on this work, cascade models of the dynamic links among risk and protective factors have sought to integrate findings. These sophisticated models will provide critical information to advance theoretical and practical applications (Dodge et al., 2009; Sitnick et al., 2014).

Assessment and Identification in the School Context

As certain behaviors carry age restrictions (e.g., cigarette and alcohol use in the U.S.), endorsement may pose additional risk for underage users. Confidentiality, therefore, is a critical component of accurate assessment. Data suggest that adolescents prefer, and may be more truthful in responding to, paper and computerized questionnaires as compared to interviews with adults (e.g., nurses, teachers; Knight et al., 2007). Further, although self report is the most common, inexpensive, and minimally invasive manner of ascertaining substance use, findings remain mixed in regard to accuracy at the individual level (e.g., Williams & Nowatzki, 2005). Finally, changes in substance use disorder criteria made in the DSM-5 (American Psychiatric Association, 2013) could impact risk-related assessments, (e.g., removal of recurrent legal problems); to date, no DSM-5 symptom-derived assessments for youth have been published.

With these considerations in mind, the YRBSS and MTF questionnaires are publicly available, and thus allow for the incorporation of standardized questions (e.g., "have you ever used . . ." and "in the past 30 days . . .") in regard to prevalence and frequency of alcohol, cigarette, and marijuana use as well as broad-based risk assessment (e.g., age of initiation; binge drinking frequency). The Adolescent Alcohol and Drug Involvement Scale (AADIS; Moberg, 2000) is another, relatively brief, self-report assessment of frequency of use across a wider variety of substance use categories. This face-valid measure, successfully used in clinical and community-based samples (e.g., Blumenthal et al., 2011), asks youth to select a single answer on a 0 (*never used*) to 7 (*several times a day*) scale that best reflects typical use of the identified substance. The CRAFFT (an acronym based on the six questions; Knight, Sherritt, Shrier, Harris, & Chang, 2002) is the most widely studied adolescent substance use risk screener (Stewart & Connors, 2004). This instrument is easy to score and provides an estimated risk level (i.e. low, medium, high). In terms of alcohol use specifically, the Alcohol Use Disorders Identification Test (AUDIT; Saunders, Aasland, Babor, De la Fuente, & Grant 1993) also has been extensively employed in adolescent samples (e.g., Chung et al., 2000). The AUDIT includes 10 questions on overall alcohol use as well as problems reflecting selected DSM-IV criteria for alcohol abuse and dependence.

Finally, incorporation of assessments of factors related to subsequent substance use risk may aid in early identification as well as appropriate intervention enrollment. Although certain substance-specific motives are missing, adaptations of the Drinking Motives Questionnaire-Revised (Cooper, 1994) have been successfully employed in adolescent cigarette and marijuana assessments (e.g., Comeau, Stewart, & Loba, 2001). Further, the Substance Use Risk Profile Scale (SURPS; Woicik, Stewart, Pihl, & Conrod, 2009) was designed for the assessment of substance-related risk among youth (e.g., sensation seeking).

Compared to work conducted with adults, validation of measures for use with children and adolescents has received less attention. Continued efforts in the design and testing of materials targeting youth is important given: (1) limited utility of lifetime and 'current' (e.g., past 30-day) history in capturing those at risk for substance use problems, and (2) distinctions in youth experience and reporting (e.g., Chen & Anthony, 2003) of related problems as compared to adults. Further, the standardized use of reliable, well-validated screening and assessment procedures will aid in both the application and evaluation of school-based intervention programs.

Evidence-based Interventions

Over the past two decades alone, hundreds of articles have been published reporting school-based substance use intervention development and outcomes, reviews and meta-analyses of such programs (e.g., Cuijpers, 2002; Wagner et al., 2004), reviews of reviews (Flay, 2009), and analyses of meta-analyses (Sandler et al., 2014). The following section will present general findings regarding consistent facets of universal approaches (e.g., general information, social influence, inter/intrapersonal competence), characteristics that cut across approaches and programs (e.g., non-interactive or interactive), as well as briefly outline three promising programs that stand out in this extensive literature: one universal program based in the U.S. (*LifeSkills Training;* Botvin, Griffin, Diaz, & Ifill-Williams, 2001), one universal program in Europe (*Unplugged*; Faggiano et al., 2007), and one selective personality-targeted program (*PreVenture*; Conrod, Stewart, Comeau, & Maclean, 2006) with replicated and extended data collected in Canada and the U.K.

Information regarding the acute and long-term effects of substance use is a key feature of intervention; however, universal prevention programs focused *primarily* on the provision of knowledge evidence minimal short-term benefit at best, and in some cases correlate with subsequent increases in substance use (see Botvin & Griffin, 2007; Faggiano et al., 2008; Flay, 2009; Lemstra et al., 2010 for exemplar reviews). In addition to fidelity concerns, such efforts may overlook key developmental considerations, such as responsivity to, and encoding of, experienced reward and punishment events (see Albert & Steinberg, 2011). Conversely, programs focusing on social influence (e.g., explicit/implicit influences, normative data) and/or competence (e.g., general problem solving, stress management) are clearly grounded in the developmental context and risk-related phenomena (e.g., perceptions of attitudes, maturation of affect regulation systems). Collectively, such programs evidence small but significant effects on the incidence and progression of substance use (Faggiano et al., 2008; Hwang, Yeagley, & Petosa, 2004; Porath-Waller, Beasley, & Beirness, 2010), although individual program findings are heterogeneous.

Closer examination reveals several key characteristics, or 'ingredients' (Cuijpers, 2002) that distinguish the more effective programs within larger literature. For example, interactive programs (as opposed to simply providing normative, affective, or skill-based information) were most effective in terms of behavioral outcomes (Faggiano et al., 2008; Porath-Waller et al., 2010; Tobler et al., 2000). Utilization of non-teacher leaders (e.g., clinicians, older adolescents) was associated with better outcomes (Gottfredson & Wilson, 2003; Tobler et al., 2000), as was the inclusion of multiple methods (Hwang et al., 2004; Lemstra et al., 2010), and regular fidelity checks (Porath-Waller et al., 2010). Although several studies indicate that extended programs and/or 'booster' sessions are beneficial (Tobler et al., 2000), findings are not consistent, and likely differ as a function of other program components (Cuijpers, 2002). Finally, Hwang and colleagues' (2004) analysis found that smoking interventions categorized as cognitive behavioral (as opposed to purely social influence or skill-based) evidenced the largest effect sizes. Further efforts examining intervention content, as well as generalizability across substances, are needed.

LifeSkills Training

LifeSkills Training (LST) is the most rigorously tested universal school substance use prevention program in the U.S. (see http://www.lifeskillstraining.com/index.php for LST materials, research, and additional resources). Classified as a Top Tier program by the Coalition for Evidence-Based Policy, an extensive literature indicates that this comparatively low-cost program effectively reduces the initiation and frequency of use across multiple substances (e.g., Botvin & Griffin, 2002; Griffin, Botvin, Nichols, & Doyle, 2003). This program utilizes a cognitive behavioral approach to social influence and competence enhancement targets (e.g., via rehearsal, reinforcement, and homework assignments), including challenging common misconceptions regarding substance use, general problem analysis and decision-making, as well as verbal and nonverbal communication and assertiveness skills. Although the middle school program implemented by trained teachers is the most extensively studied, curricula have been developed for elementary and high school students, data indicate successful provision via trained counselors and other professionals, and complementary parent support and violence prevention modules may be incorporated.

Unplugged

Unplugged is the first comprehensive universal school-based substance use program subject to systematic testing in Europe (see http://www.eudap.net/Home.aspx for *Unplugged* materials, research, and additional resources). Tailored to European school systems, a growing literature supports short-term efficacy (e.g., reducing alcohol, cigarette, and marijuana use three months after program completion), as well as reductions in the frequency and amount of alcohol and marijuana use at a 15-month follow-up (e.g., Faggiano et al., 2010). The program draws from both behavioral and health models, targeting social influence and competence via units including substance use knowledge and normative beliefs, critical thinking and decision-making, coping with emotions and stress, as well as communication and relationship skills. Currently, *Unplugged* is designed for teacher provision to students ages 12–14 years; although peer and parent components have been developed, preliminary data do not indicate any additional benefit (Faggiano et al., 2010). All materials are freely available online (although provider training is strongly suggested), and data regarding program expansion (e.g., location), potential moderators (e.g., sex, socio-economic status) and mediators (e.g., appraisal of norms, interpersonal skills) are rapidly being disseminated.

PreVenture

PreVenture is the only evidence-based selective school substance use intervention program in Canada and the U.K.; additional location (e.g., Czech Republic, Australia) as well as culturally grounded (e.g., Mi'kmaq First Nations communities in Nova Scotia, Canada) adaptations are underway (see http://co-venture.ca/en/ for general information, research, and additional resources). A number of randomized controlled trials indicate short- and long-term reductions in the initiation and risk-related use of alcohol (e.g., binge drinking; coping-motivated; Conrod et al., 2013), and a growing literature provides support for the program in preventing or reducing other substance use (e.g., Conrod, Castellanos-Ryan, & Strang, 2010) as well as relevant psychological problems (e.g., depression; Castellanos, & Conrod, 2006). Following a screening for four targeted personality dimensions (anxiety sensitivity, hopelessness, impulsivity, sensation seeking), tailored intervention modules integrate psychoeducation, motivational enhancement, and cognitive behavioral approaches. Components of the intervention are fitted to the identified characteristic (e.g., hopelessness/negative thinking), and include psychoeducation on the specified trait and associated behaviors (e.g., avoidance, substance misuse), goal setting, structured discussion of personal experiences, identification of triggers, and challenging cognitive distortions. Current reports support implementation of the program with youth ages 13 years and older, and preliminary effectiveness studies indicate that delivery by trained teachers is comparable to the majority of trials which included masters-level clinician facilitators (O'Leary-Barrett, Mackie, Castellanos-Ryan, Al-Khudhairy, & Conrod, 2010).

Cultural, Social, and Contextual Considerations

Increasingly, developmental and prevention scientists have sought to understand widely studied microsystem-level risk (e.g., individual difference factors, familial and peer influence) in the larger context of structural, environmental, and psychological aspects of local communities and national culture. Henggler, Schoenwald, Borduin, Rowland, and Cunningham's (2009) Multisystemic Therapy, for example, recognizes the need to intervene at multiple levels (i.e., individual, familial, peers, school, and neighborhood) to reduce youth antisocial behavior, including substance use. Availability of community-level supports, such as organized service groups and activity clubs, not only are linked with concurrent and prospective declines in adolescent substance use (Eccles, Barber, Stone, & Hunt 2003), but also have been found to significantly impact the positive effects of school-based programming (Cuijpers, 2002; Hwang et al., 2004; Tobler et al., 2000). Further, community-based efforts, including comprehensive training of purveyors of alcohol and cigarettes, compliance checks of age-appropriate sales, and establishment of local ordinances supporting such efforts (e.g., mandating training, penalization of failure to check for age identification) reduce access to alcohol and cigarettes among older teens, and may bolster the effects of concurrent school-based programs (e.g., *Project Northland*; Perry et al., 2002).

Several programs evidence success across diverse racial, ethnic, and cultural samples; however, limited work has compared these programs to that which has been culturally grounded. Cultural grounding, which may include both surface (e.g., adapting images, name and location references) and deep (e.g., incorporation of cultural values) targeting, may enhance youth 'buy in' and internalization of program messages. For example, factors such as racial discrimination (Gibbons et al., 2012) and acculturation (Schwartz, Unger, Zamboanga, & Szapocznik, 2010) each have been linked to substance use risk, and thus may be important components of relevant intervention efforts. Operationalizing group membership and targets requires great care, both in terms of monitoring potential biases and stereotypes as well as considering the multifaceted nature of identity (e.g., intersectionality; Unger 2012). The use of participatory research approaches will be key to building the components of targeted designs (e.g., Perry et al., 2002). Colby and colleagues (2013) present an exceptional review of the processes and pitfalls experienced in their adaptation of the *keepin it REAL* program for use with a rural population.

Take-Home Points

- Despite concerted efforts, substance use among adolescents remains a problem, and the use of alternative uptake (e.g., e-cigarettes) and unregulated substances requires further study.
- Multiple factors are identified in developmentally informed models of youth substance use, including genetic and neurological correlates, cognitions, and personality factors, as well as familial and peer behaviors and attitudes.
- Maintaining confidentiality is an important consideration when dealing with self-reported illicit behavior.
- Key features of effective school-based substance use interventions include interaction, multiple methods, and regular fidelity checks. Education about the effects of substance use may be a necessary, but insufficient, ingredient for intervention programs.
- Programs that focus on developmentally appropriate considerations display promising effects on reducing the onset and harmful progression of substance use.
- Community organizations and community-based efforts can be important components of intervention, being related to decreased substance use and the potential to increase the effect of school-based substance use programs.
- Evidence-based programs have evidenced effectiveness across many groups. However, research on culturally adapted or culturally targeted interventions is limited.

Resources

Commonly used assessment measures include:

- YRBSS (http://www.cdc.gov/healthyyouth/data/yrbs/data.htm) and MTF (http://www.icpsr.umich.edu/icpsrweb/SAMHDA/series/35) questionnaires
- CRAAFT (Knight et al., 2002)
- Substance Use Risk Profile Scale (SURPS; Woicik et al., 2009)
- Example school-based substance use intervention programs include:
- *LifeSkills Training* (Universal; see http://www.lifeskillstraining.com/index.php)
- *Unplugged* (Universal; see http://www.eudap.net/Home.aspx)
- *PreVenture* (Selective, personality targeted; see http://co-venture.ca/en/)
- See also http://toptierevidence.org/ and http://www.samhsa.gov/ebp-web-guide/substance-abuse-prevention for additional information on available evidence-based programming and resources

References

Albert, D., & Steinberg, L. (2011). Judgment and decision making in adolescence. *Journal of Research on Adolescence, 21*, 211–224. doi: 10.1111/j.1532–7795.2010.00724.x

American Psychiatric Association (APA). (2013). *Diagnostic and statistical manual of mental disorders* (5th ed.) (DSM-5). Washington, DC: American Psychiatric Association.

Blumenthal, H., Leen-Feldner, E.W., Badour, C.L., & Babson, K.A. (2011). Anxiety psychopathology and alcohol use among adolescents: A critical review of the empirical literature and recommendations for future research. *Journal of Experimental Psychopathology, 2*, 318–353. doi: 10.5127/jep.012810

Botvin, G.J., & Griffin, K.W. (2002). Life skills training as a primary prevention approach for adolescent drug abuse and other problem behaviors. *International Journal of Emergency Mental Health, 4*, 41–48.

Botvin, G.J., & Griffin, K.W. (2007). School-based programmes to prevent alcohol, tobacco and other drug use. *International Review of Psychiatry, 19*, 607–615. doi: 10.1080/09540260701797753

Botvin, G.J., Griffin, K.W., Diaz, T., & Ifill-Williams, M. (2001). Drug abuse prevention among minority adolescents: Posttest and one-year follow-up of a school-based preventive intervention. *Prevention Science, 2*, 1–13. doi: 10.1023/A:1010025311161

Brown, S.A., McGue, M., Maggs, J., Schulenberg, J., Hingson, R., Swartzwelder, S., . . . Murphy, S. (2008). A developmental perspective on alcohol and youths 16 to 20 years of age. *Pediatrics, 121*, S290–S310. doi: 10.1542/peds.2007–2243D

Bryant, A.L., Schulenberg, J.E., O'Malley, P.M., Bachman, J.G., & Johnston, L.D. (2003). How academic achievement, attitudes, and behaviors relate to the course of substance use during adolescence: A 6-year, multiwave national longitudinal study. *Journal of Research on Adolescence, 13*, 361–397. doi: 10.1111/1532–7795.1303005

Castellanos, N., & Conrod, P. (2006). Brief interventions targeting personality risk factors for adolescent substance misuse reduce depression, panic and risk-taking behaviours. *Journal of Mental Health, 15*, 645–658. doi: 10.1080/09638230600998912

Centers for Disease Control and Prevention (CDC). (2014). Surveillance and Evaluation Data Resources for Comprehensive Tobacco Control Programs. Atlanta, GA: Centers for Disease Control and Prevention, National Center for Chronic Disease Prevention and Health Promotion.

Chen, C.Y., & Anthony, J.C. (2003). Possible age-associated bias in reporting of clinical features of drug dependence: epidemiological evidence on adolescent-onset marijuana use. *Addiction, 98*, 71–82. doi: 10.1046/j.1360–0443.2003.00237.x

Chung, T., Colby, S.M., Barnett, N.P., Rohsenow, D.J., Spirito, A., & Monti, P.M. (2000). Screening adolescents for problem drinking: performance of brief screens against DSM-IV alcohol diagnoses. *Journal of Studies on Alcohol, 61*, 579–587.

Colby, M., Hecht, M.L., Miller-Day, M., Krieger, J.L., Syvertsen, A.K., Graham, J.W., & Pettigrew, J. (2013). Adapting school-based substance use prevention curriculum through cultural grounding: A review and exemplar of adaptation processes for rural schools. *American Journal of Community Psychology, 51*, 190–205. doi: 10.1007/s10464–012–9524–8

Comeau, N., Stewart, S.H., & Loba, P. (2001). The relations of trait anxiety, anxiety sensitivity, and sensation seeking to adolescents' motivations for alcohol, cigarette, and marijuana use. *Addictive Behaviors, 26*, 803–825. doi: 10.1016/S0306–4603(01)00238–6

Conrod, P.J., Castellanos-Ryan, N., & Strang, J. (2010). Brief, personality-targeted coping skills interventions and survival as a non–drug user over a 2-year period during adolescence. *Archives of General Psychiatry, 67*, 85–93.

Conrod, P.J., O'Leary-Barrett, M., Newton, N., Topper, L., Castellanos-Ryan, N., Mackie, C., & Girard, A. (2013). Effectiveness of a selective, personality-targeted prevention program for adolescent alcohol use and misuse: a cluster randomized controlled trial. *JAMA Psychiatry, 70,* 334–342. doi: 10.1001/jamapsychiatry.2013.651

Conrod, P.J., Stewart, S.H., Comeau, N., & Maclean, A.M. (2006). Efficacy of cognitive–behavioral interventions targeting personality risk factors for youth alcohol misuse. *Journal of Clinical Child & Adolescent Psychology, 35,* 550–563. doi: 10.1207/s15374424jccp3504_6

Cooper, M.L. (1994). Motivations for alcohol use among adolescents: Development and validation of a four-factor model. *Psychological Assessment, 6,* 117–128. doi: 10.1037/1040–3590.6.2.117

Cuijpers, P. (2002). Effective ingredients of school-based drug prevention programs: A systematic review. *Addictive Behaviors, 27,* 1009–1023. doi: 10.1016/S0306–4603(02)00295–2

Dawes, M.A., Antelman, S.M., Vanyukov, M.M., Giancola, P., Tarter, R.E., Susman, E.J., . . . & Clark, D.B. (2000). Developmental sources of variation in liability to adolescent substance use disorders. *Drug and Alcohol Dependence, 61,* 3–14. doi: 10.1016/S0376–8716(00)00120–4

Deas, D., Riggs, P., Langenbucher, J., Goldman, M., & Brown, S. (2000). Adolescents are not adults: Developmental considerations in alcohol users. *Alcoholism: Clinical and Experimental Research, 24,* 232–237. doi: 10.1111/j.1530–0277.2000.tb04596.x

Dodge, K.A., Malone, P.S., Lansford, J.E., Miller, S., Pettit, G.S., & Bates, J.E. (2009). A dynamic cascade model of the development of substance-use onset. *Monographs of the Society for Research in Child Development, 74.* doi: 10.1111/j.1540–5834.2009.00528.x

Eccles, J.S., Barber, B.L., Stone, M., & Hunt, J. (2003). Extracurricular activities and adolescent development. *Journal of Social Issues, 59,* 865–889.

Faggiano, F., Richardson, C., Bohrn, K., Galanti, M.R., & EU-Dap Study Group. (2007). A cluster randomized controlled trial of school-based prevention of tobacco, alcohol and drug use: The EU-Dap design and study population. *Preventive Medicine, 44,* 170–173.

Faggiano, F., Vigna-Taglianti, F., Burkhart, G., Bohrn, K., Cuomo, L., Gregori, D., . . . & EU-Dap Study Group. (2010). The effectiveness of a school-based substance abuse prevention program: 18-month follow-up of the EU-Dap cluster randomized controlled trial. *Drug and Alcohol Dependence, 108,* 56–64.

Faggiano, F., Vigna-Taglianti, F.D., Versino, E., Zambon, A., Borraccino, A., & Lemma, P. (2008). School-based prevention for illicit drugs use: A systematic review. *Preventive Medicine, 46,* 385–396. doi: 10.1016/j.ypmed.2007.11.012

Flay, B.R. (2009). The promise of long-term effectiveness of school-based smoking prevention programs: A critical review of reviews. *Tobacco Induced Diseases, 5,* 7. doi: 10.1186/1617–9625–5–7

Gibbons, F.X., O'Hara, R.E., Stock, M.L., Gerrard, M., Weng, C.Y., & Wills, T.A. (2012). The erosive effects of racism: reduced self-control mediates the relation between perceived racial discrimination and substance use in African American adolescents. *Journal of Personality & Social Psychology, 102,* 1089–1104. doi: 10.1037/a0027404

Gottfredson, D.C., & Wilson, D.B. (2003). Characteristics of effective school-based substance abuse prevention. *Prevention Science, 4,* 27–38. doi: 10.1023/A:1021782710278

Griffin, K.W., Botvin, G.J., Nichols, T.R., & Doyle, M.M. (2003). Effectiveness of a universal drug abuse prevention approach for youth at high risk for substance use initiation. *Preventive Medicine, 36,* 1–7.

Henggler, S.W., Schoenwald, S.K., Borduin, C.M., Rowland, M. D, & Cunningham, P.B. (2009). *Multisystemic Therapy for antisocial behavior in children and adolescents* (2nd ed.). New York: Guilford.

Hwang, M.S., Yeagley, K.L., & Petosa, R. (2004). A meta-analysis of adolescent psychosocial smoking prevention programs published between 1978 and 1997 in the United States. *Health Education & Behavior, 31*, 702–719. doi: 10.1177/1090198104263361

James, J.E., Kristjánsson, Á.L., & Sigfúsdóttir, I.D. (2011). Adolescent substance use, sleep, and academic achievement: Evidence of harm due to caffeine. *Journal of Adolescence, 34*, 665–673. doi: 10.1016/j.adolescence.2010.09.006

Jeynes, W.H. (2002). The relationship between the consumption of various drugs by adolescents and their academic achievement. *The American Journal of Drug & Alcohol Abuse, 28*, 15–35.

Johnston, L.D., O'Malley, P.M., Miech, R.A., Bachman, J.G., & Schulenberg, J.E. (2015). *Monitoring the Future national survey results on drug use: 1975–2014: Overview, key findings on adolescent drug use.* Ann Arbor: Institute for Social Research.

Kann, L., Kinchen, S., Shanklin, S.L., Flint, K.H., Hawkins, J., . . . & Zaza, S. (2014). *Morbidity and Mortality Weekly Report 2014, 63*, SS-4. Retrieved from http://www.cdc.gov/healthyyouth/data/yrbs/results.htm

Knight, J.R., Harris, S.K., Sherritt, L., Van Hook, S., Lawrence, N., Brooks, T., Carey, P., Kossack, R., & Kulig, J. (2007). Adolescents' preference for substance abuse screening in primary care practice. *Substance Abuse, 28*, 107–117. doi: 10.1300/J465v28n04_03

Knight, J.R., Sherritt, L., Shrier, L.A., Harris, S.K., & Chang, G. (2002). Validity of the CRAFFT substance abuse screening test among adolescent clinic patients. *Archives of Pediatrics & Adolescent Medicine, 156*, 607–614. doi: 10.1001/archpedi.156.6.607

Lemstra, M., Bennett, N., Nannapaneni, U., Neudorf, C., Warren, L., Kershaw, T., & Scott, C. (2010). A systematic review of school-based marijuana and alcohol prevention programs targeting adolescents aged 10–15. *Addiction Research & Theory, 18*, 84–96.

Miller, T.R., Levy, D.T., Spicer, R.S., & Taylor, D. (2006). Societal costs of underage drinking. *Journal of Studies on Alcohol, 57*, 519–528.

Moberg, D.P. (2000). The Adolescent Alcohol and Drug Involvement Scale: An instrument for measuring adolescent use and misuse of alcohol. *Journal of Studies on Alcohol, 40*, 291–300.

O'Leary-Barrett, M., Mackie, C.J., Castellanos-Ryan, N., Al-Khudhairy, N., & Conrod, P.J. (2010). Personality-targeted interventions delay uptake of drinking and decrease risk of alcohol-related problems when delivered by teachers. *Journal of the American Academy of Child & Adolescent Psychiatry, 49*, 954–963. doi: 10.1016/j.jaac.2010.04.011

Perry, C.L., Williams, C.L., Komro, K.A., Veblen-Mortenson, S., Stigler, M.H., Munson, K.A., . . . & Forster, J.L. (2002). Project Northland: Long-term outcomes of community action to reduce adolescent alcohol use. *Health Education Research, 17*, 117–132. doi: 10.1093/her/17.1.117

Porath-Waller, A.J., Beasley, E., & Beirness, D.J. (2010). A meta-analytic review of school-based prevention for cannabis use. *Health Education & Behavior.* Online First. doi: 10.1177/1090198110361315

Roebuck, M.C., French, M.T., & Dennis, M.L. (2004). Adolescent marijuana use and school attendance. *Economics of Education Review, 23*, 133–141. doi: 10.1016/S0272–7757(03)00079–7

Sandler, I., Wolchik, S.A., Cruden, G., Mahrer, N.E., Ahn, S., Brincks, A., & Brown, C.H. (2014). Overview of meta-analyses of the prevention of mental health, substance use, and conduct problems. *Annual Review of Clinical Psychology, 10*, 243–273. doi: 10.1146/annurev-clinpsy-050212–185524

Saraceno, L., Munafó, M., Heron, J., Craddock, N., & van den Bree, M.B.M. (2009). Genetic and non-genetic influences on the development of co-occurring alcohol problem use and internalizing symptomatology in adolescence: A review. *Addiction, 104*, 1100–1121. doi: 10.1111/j.1360–0443.2009.02571.x

Sargent, J.D., Tanski, S., Stoolmiller, M., & Hanewinkel, R. (2010). Using sensation seeking to target adolescents for substance use interventions. *Addiction, 105*, 506–514. doi: 10.1111/j.1360–0443.2009.02782.x

Saunders, J.B., Aasland, O.G., Babor, T.F., De la Fuente, J.R., & Grant, M. (1993). Development of the alcohol use disorders identification test (AUDIT): WHO collaborative project on early detection of persons with harmful alcohol consumption-II. *Addiction, 88*, 791–804.

Schwartz, S.J., Unger, J.B., Zamboanga, B.L., & Szapocznik, J. (2010). Rethinking the concept of acculturation: Implications for theory and research. *American Psychologist, 65*, 237–251. doi: 10.1037/a0019330

Sher, K.J., Bartholow, B.D., & Wood, M.D. (2000). Personality and substance use disorders: a prospective study. *Journal of Consulting and Clinical Psychology, 68*, 818–829. doi: 10.1037/0022–006X.68.5.818

Sitnick, S.L., Shaw, D.S., & Hyde, L.W. (2014). Precursors of adolescent substance use from early childhood and early adolescence: Testing a developmental cascade model. *Development and Psychopathology, 26*, 125–140. doi: 10.1017/S0954579413000539

Squeglia, L.M., Jacobus, J., & Tapert, S.F. (2009). The influence of substance use on adolescent brain development. *Clinical EEG and Neuroscience, 40*, 31–38.

Stewart, S.H., & Connors, G.J. (2004) Screening for alcohol problems: What makes a test effective? *Alcohol Research & Health, 28*, 5–16.

Tobler, N.S., Roona, M.R., Ochshorn, P., Marshall, D.G., Streke, A.V., & Stackpole, K.M. (2000). School-based adolescent drug prevention programs: 1998 meta-analysis. *Journal of Primary Prevention, 20*, 275–336. doi: 10.1023/A:1021314704811

Townsend, L., Flisher, A.J., & King, G. (2007). A systematic review of the relationship between high school dropout and substance use. *Clinical Child and Family Psychology Review, 10*, 295–317. doi: 10.1007/s10567–007–0023–7

Unger, J.B. (2012). The most critical unresolved issues associated with race, ethnicity, culture, and substance use. *Substance Use & Misuse, 47*, 390–395. doi: 10.3109/10826084.2011.638017

Wagner, E.F., Tubman, J.G., & Gil, A.G. (2004). Implementing school-based abuse interventions: Methodological dilemmas and recommended solutions. *Addiction, 99*, 106–119. doi: 10.1111/j.1360–0443.2004.00858.x

Williams, R.J., & Nowatzki, N. (2005). Validity of adolescent self-report of substance use. *Substance Use & Misuse, 40*, 299–311. doi: 10.1081/JA-200049327

Windle, M. (2000). Parental, sibling, and peer influences on adolescent substance use and alcohol problems. *Applied Developmental Science, 4*, 98–110. doi: 10.1207/S1532480XADS0402_5

Windle, M., Spear, L.P., Fuligni, A.J., Angold, A., Brown, J.D., Pine, D., . . . & Dahl, R.E. (2008). Transitions into underage and problem drinking: developmental processes and mechanisms between 10 and 15 years of age. *Pediatrics, 121*, S273–S289. doi: 10.1542/peds.2007–2243C

Wittchen, H.U., Fröhlich, C., Behrendt, S., Günther, A., Rehm, J., Zimmermann, P., . . . & Perkonigg, A. (2007). Cannabis use and cannabis use disorders and their relationship to mental disorders: A 10-year prospective-longitudinal community study in adolescents. *Drug and Alcohol Dependence, 88*, S60–S70. doi: 10.1016/j.drugalcdep.2006.12.013

Woicik, P.A., Stewart, S.H., Pihl, R.O., & Conrod, P.J. (2009). The substance use risk profile scale: A scale measuring traits linked to reinforcement-specific substance use profiles. *Addictive Behaviors, 34*, 1042–1055. doi: 10.1016/j.addbeh.2009.07.001

7

ADOLESCENT EATING DISORDERS AND OBESITY

Stuart B. Murray, Andrea B. Goldschmidt, and Daniel Le Grange

Eating disorders continue to rank amongst the most serious and damaging of all psychiatric disorders, and have for many years posed significant challenges for both patients and their families alike. Although the precise etiology of eating disorders is unknown, their multifactorial impact, which spans social, psychological, neurological and biological processes, has made effective treatment an elusive goal, and current leading treatment approaches are generally thought of as falling short of acceptable treatment outcomes as compared to other psychiatric conditions (Bulik, Berkman, Brownley, Sedway, & Lohr, 2007). Further compounding the complexities of effective treatment, the risk of non-effective treatment far outweighs the risk encountered in many other psychiatric conditions. For instance, in assessing the physiological and psychosocial consequences of eating disorders, research demonstrates frequent and severe medical complications with mortality rates of up to 20% (Steinhausen, 2002), vastly elevated rates of suicidality (Pompili, Mancinelli, Girardi, Ruberto, & Tatarelli, 2004), impaired quality of life (Mond, Hay, Rodgers, Owen, & Beumont, 2005), and a chronic and relapsing illness course (Treasure & Russell, 2011). Indeed, in glancing back over the recent history of the treatment of eating disorders, poor rates of full symptom remission (Steinhausen, 2002), high rates of transdiagnostic crossover between eating disorder diagnoses (Eddy et al., 2008), and high rates of relapse abound (Keel & Brown, 2010). Thus, the effective treatment of eating disorders remains of crucial importance.

With particular respect to eating disorders during adolescence, the importance of enhancing treatment outcomes in this population group is heavily underscored by findings demonstrating that eating disorders most commonly emerge during the course of adolescence (Kohn & Golden, 2001) and are most rapidly increasing in adolescents (Smink, van Hoeken & Hoek, 2012). Furthermore, robust findings also demonstrate that the most favorable treatment outcomes appear to coincide with earlier points of treatment intervention (Rome et al., 2003), with anorexia nervosa treated in adolescence being characterized by lower mortality rates, reduced illness chronicity, and greater rates of recovery and symptom improvement (Steinhausen, 2002) than when treated in adulthood. However, despite such findings, the relative weighting of research and treatment studies still leans towards adult presentations of eating disorders, although the last decade has witnessed a surge in treatment studies investigating adolescent eating disorders. In this chapter, we will aim to summarize emerging research pertaining to the distinct profiles of disordered eating, the prevalence of adolescent eating disorders, their treatment, and the socio-ecological context in which adolescent eating disorders are maintained.

Differing Types of Eating Disorders in Adolescence

Anorexia Nervosa

Anorexia nervosa (AN) is a serious mental illness, which is most centrally characterized by an unrelenting pursuit of thinness; a failure to maintain a minimally normal body weight; and intense preoccupations around food, weight, and shape. Whilst AN currently affects up to 1% of the population, evidence suggests that the prevalence is increasing (Attia, 2010), with the most common age of onset falling within adolescence (Kohn & Golden, 2001). Presentations of AN take one of two subtypes: AN-restricting and AN-binge/purge subtype. This distinction helps delineate those with AN who solely reduce their food intake from those whose behaviors include compensatory purging (i.e., vomiting, compulsive exercise, the use of diuretics and laxatives), with or without sporadic episodes of binge eating (Attia, 2010). Recent changes in diagnostic criteria have relaxed strict criteria regarding the use of a specific body weight as a diagnostic marker, and have also removed amenorrhea as a diagnostic marker (APA, 2013). This may have specific implications for pre-adolescent youth and boys, who may now be more accurately diagnosed with AN.

Bulimia Nervosa

Bulimia nervosa (BN) is most centrally characterized by recurrent episodes of binge eating, in which the adolescent consumes an atypically large volume of food in a discrete period of time while experiencing a sense of loss of control. Alongside such episodes, compensatory behaviors undertaken to offset possible weight gain include self-induced vomiting, laxative abuse, dietary restriction, and compulsive exercise. A pervasive overvaluation of shape and weight maintains symptomatology, although high degrees of guilt and shame may often make symptom detection difficult, particularly given that most BN patients do not present as underweight. Although the prevalence of BN is approximately 1% of the population (Swanson, Crow, Le Grange, Swendson, & Merikangas, 2011), it is likely that the prevalence may increase in light of the diagnostic criteria reducing the strict yet arbitrary binge frequency criterion (APA, 2013).

Binge Eating Disorder

Binge eating disorder (BED) is defined by recurrent episodes of binge eating that are not accompanied by the regular use of inappropriate compensatory behaviors seen in BN. Binge eating episodes are associated with marked distress and are often characterized by eating much more rapidly than usual; eating when not physically hungry; eating alone due to embarrassment; eating until uncomfortably full; and feeling ashamed, embarrassed, or very guilty. Unlike AN and BN, body image disturbance is not currently included among the criteria for BED, although there is some evidence that overvaluation of shape and weight may be a useful diagnostic specifier for the disorder given its significance as an indicator of illness severity and treatment outcome (e.g., Goldschmidt et al., 2008; Grilo, 2013). BED affects approximately 1–2% of community-based adolescents (Swanson et al., 2011), but this prevalence rate does not reflect the relatively high frequency with which adolescents report subthreshold binge eating behaviors that fail to the meet the size or frequency threshold required for a diagnosis of BED, but nevertheless cause significant distress and impairment (Johnson, Rohan, & Kirk, 2002; Neumark-Sztainer, Wall, Larson, Eisenberg, & Loth, 2011).

How School Personnel Might Assist

In identifying students at risk or suffering from eating disorders, school personnel may play a significant role in both identifying early illness sequelae and facilitating pathways to treatment. For instance, early signs of AN typically involve the exclusion of particular food groups, the development of rigid food rules, driven exercise, increased efforts at concealing one's body, and, perhaps most ostensibly, rapid weight loss. In the case of BN, early warning signs feature an array of discernable symptoms, including periodic episodes of eating large volumes of food interspersed with episodes of restrictive eating, frequent attempts purging following the consumption of meals, attempts at secretive eating, driven exercise, and laxative use. Early warning signs for BED may similarly include periodic episodes of eating large quantities of food and eating secretively, in addition to large and/or rapid changes in body weight.

In noting any of these features in students, we would advise that school personnel act swiftly, given that the earlier point at which treatment can be administered often relates to more favorable treatment outcomes (Treasure & Russell, 2011). However, since eating disorders are often inclusive of internalized guilt and shame, any potential screening conversation should be cautiously undertaken by a school counselor or somebody with mental health training. In light of the medical complications of untreated eating disorders, and since most evidence-based treatments for adolescent eating disorders feature some degree of parental involvement, we would recommend that school personnel share any concerns and observations with parents and provide information outlining how to obtain a more rigorous assessment by trained specialists.

It is possible that throughout the course of treatment, students with eating disorders will be required to take time off school to access intensive treatment. As such, school counseling staff may assist in liaising between the expectations of the school and curriculum and those of the treatment program, with many intensive programs requesting school work for adolescents as they undergo treatment. Furthermore, upon being discharged from intensive treatment facilities, the reintegration back to school may be challenging for many reasons. For instance, adolescents often report anxiety around what to tell friends and teachers in explaining their absence from school. Additionally, social eating with friends at lunch and recess can be exceedingly challenging, and some may require extra support from counseling staff or parents during meals. During the reintegration of students back into school settings, close liaison between school staff, treating clinicians, and parents should be coordinated in carefully outlining the optimal role for school staff.

Summary of School Personnel Involvement

- Be familiar with the various types of eating disorders and their early warning signs.
- Be prepared to act swiftly when being made aware of any symptoms.
- Approach any screening conversation cautiously.
- Feedback your concerns to parents and offer avenues for a professional assessment.
- Continue to liaise with treatment team and parents throughout treatment.
- Liaise with school staff in adjusting academic expectations, if necessary, and also provide core curriculum work to student if their treatment program permits.
- Be prepared to be actively involved in the reintegration of students into school life and liaise with treating clinicians and parents in determining the optimal role.

Evidence-based Treatment for Eating Disorders in Adolescence

Anorexia Nervosa

Inpatient treatment. Current evidence suggests enhanced treatment outcomes when the length of inpatient admissions are reduced to focus on strict medical stabilization, as opposed to focusing on weight restoration, which takes significantly longer (Madden et al., 2015). Additionally, many have documented the detrimental psychosocial consequences of in-patient admissions for adolescents during important developmental stages (Gowers & Bryant-Waugh, 2004; Gowers et al., 2007). Thus, although the need exists for inpatient medical stabilization in acute instances, limited inpatient admissions and a rapid transition to outpatient treatment appears to promote favorable treatment outcomes.

Family-based treatment. The family-based treatment (FBT) of adolescent AN may be characterized by an agnostic stance towards the origin of AN, alongside the overarching philosophy that parents themselves are the primary and most effective resource in their child's recovery (Lock & Le Grange, 2013). As such, FBT is oriented towards empowering parental strengths and resources in directly curtailing the behavioral symptoms of AN, in addition to ensuring nutritional rehabilitation and rapid weight restoration in their child. Initial parental efforts are oriented towards swift weight restoration, although over time and with declining symptom severity, less parental authority is typically required and the adolescent may demonstrate more autonomy over food and eating without losing weight or engaging in the behavioral symptoms of AN (Lock & Le Grange, 2013). As such, the adolescent may gradually return to normative and age-appropriate adolescent endeavors, which allows for a more central therapeutic focus on general adolescent issues away from food and eating (Lock & Le Grange, 2013).

Empirical evidence suggests that between 50 and 75% of adolescents are typically weight restored within a year of commencing FBT (Le Grange & Eisler, 2009), with 6- and 12-month follow-ups indicating that these treatment gains are robust over time (Couturier, Kimber, & Szatmari, 2013; Lock, Couturier, & Agras, 2008). In terms of the psychological symptomatology, FBT has shown a promising capacity to alleviate the cognitive and attitudinal symptomatology of AN, comparing favorably with other adolescent treatment interventions (Lock et al., 2010). However, it ought to be noted that between 30 and 50% of patients do not fully remit during FBT (Fisher, Hetrick, & Rushford, 2010), and ongoing research is warranted in further augmenting the active therapeutic processes throughout FBT.

Multi-family therapy. Multi-family therapy is an alternate family therapy-based approach to the treatment of adolescent AN, which typically unites 6–8 families in the shared and co-constructed treatment of adolescent AN. The presence of several families working alongside one another in overcoming AN cultivates strong destigmatizing processes for both parents and children alike, which facilitates empowerment and symptom remission. Furthermore, the shared forum between families allows for the experience of both being helped by other families and acting as consultants to other families, further solidifying one's own sense of efficacy and agency (Dare & Eisler, 2000).

Multi-family therapy for AN features an interchangeable use of structural, systemic, and narrative family therapy practices that are reflexively employed.

Examples of such practices may include video-recorded family meals, group feedback, 'foster family meals' in which children rotate and eat with different families, psychodrama and family sculpting practices, and psycho-educational information pertaining to the nature of eating disorders and the avoidant-based symptomatology which may emerge in attempting to avoid confronting food-based fears and anxieties (Dare & Eisler, 2000).

Controlled empirical evidence supporting multi-family therapy for AN remains sparse, although preliminary findings report that the majority of families who engage in multi-family therapy are successful in bringing about weight restoration and a stabilization in the eating practices in their child (Dare & Eisler, 2000; Scholz & Asen, 2001). Furthermore, treatment acceptability and feasibility may be inferred by low rates of treatment drop out (Dare & Eisler, 2000; Scholz & Asen, 2001). However, it should be noted that only tentative conclusions may be drawn at this stage, since the sample sizes in the few existing empirical studies have been modest. Thus, further research is warranted in illustrating the efficacy of multi-family therapy.

Adolescent-focused therapy. AFT targets the core deficits in adolescent development, which are assumed to be etiologically implicated in the adolescent's symptom presentation, through a continued clinical focus on self-exploration and the development of the 'self' (Fitzpatrick, Moye, Hoste, Lock, & Le Grange, 2010; Robin, Siegal, Koepke, Moye, & Tice, 1994; Robin et al., 1999). For instance, in presentations of AN, self-starvation and preoccupation with food and weight may often be linked to the avoidance of negative affective states associated with one's normative adolescent development, with treatment aiming to facilitate more adaptive coping styles such that one's developmental trajectory is not impaired by the use of AN as a coping strategy (Fitzpatrick et al., 2010).

Thus, the first phase of treatment is oriented towards establishing a therapeutic alliance and a preliminary understanding of the ways in which AN serves as a coping strategy for managing or avoiding challenging developmental issues. Subsequently, the second phase of AFT is oriented towards adolescent exploration of issues surrounding individuation which may have been impeded by AN, with a view towards developing age-appropriate independence from one's parents and family. Finally, the third phase of treatment is oriented towards the preparation of strategies that will lead to more sustained autonomy and independence.

To date, AFT has been the subject of a number of randomized control trials comparing several treatments for adolescent AN. Such trials have generally concluded that AFT is a viable treatment alternative to FBT in the treatment of adolescent AN, noting comparable rates of symptom remission at end-of-treatment, despite less robust long-term symptom remission for both weight- and cognitive-related symptoms (Lock et al., 2010).

Cognitive behavioral therapy. Cognitive behavioral therapy (CBT) typically consists of therapeutic interventions that aim to modify irrational cognitions and assist in the generation of disconfirmatory evidence to create cognitive dissonance between irrational thoughts and behavioral outcomes. With specific respect to eating disorders, CBT aims to restructure cognitions surrounding the over-valuation of weight and shape, in addition to modifying behaviors based on such irrational cognitions, including the development of food rules and avoidance, feared weight ranges, and compulsive exercise practices (Fairburn, 2008).

Although more commonly prescribed in the context of adult presentations of AN, recent preliminary evidence has advanced an 'enhanced' form of CBT that specifically targets the core maintaining features of eating disorder psychopathology, which was recently examined in the context of adolescent presentations of AN (Grave, Calugi, Doll, & Fairburn, 2013). Findings with adolescents reported modest rates of weight gain, with approximately 19% of those offered treatment reaching their ideal body weight by the end of treatment. However, more impressive findings were indicated by the rates of adolescents self-reporting an absence of eating disordered cognitions and behaviors by end of treatment (Grave et al., 2013), although the limitations of self-report methods of indexing psychopathology in ego-syntonic illnesses have recently been noted (Murray, Loeb, & Le Grange, 2014). Thus, further research is warranted in establishing the efficacy of CBT treatments in adolescent presentations of AN.

Psychopharmacological treatment. In examining the efficacy of psychotropic medication in directly impacting upon AN symptomatology, antidepressants, selective serotonin reuptake inhibitors (SSRI), and antipsychotic drugs have been assessed, although mixed findings have emerged so far (Balestrieri, Oriani, Simoncini, & Bellantuono, 2013). For instance, these studies report no significant differences on BMI- and cognitive-related outcomes in adolescent AN when comparing those treated with antidepressant and SSRI medication and those not treated with psychotropic medication (Balestrieri et al., 2013). Somewhat similarly, controlled trials examining antipsychotic medication showed no significant improvement in weight- and cognitive-related AN psychopathology in those treated with olanzapine as compared to those receiving placebo medication (Kafantaris et al., 2011). As such, a recent review concluded that atypical antipsychotic medications do not benefit adolescents with AN (Brandenburg, Lesser, Mangham, & Crow, 2011). This review is in accordance with a recent meta-analysis in adult AN which concluded that atypical antipsychotics do not reliably result in any weight- or cognitive-related improvements in AN symptomatology, although they do alleviate depressive symptomatology (Lebow, Sim, Erwin, & Murad, 2013).

Bulimia Nervosa

Cognitive behavioral therapy. In adult populations with BN, a wealth of empirical evidence points towards the value of cognitive behavioral therapy (CBT); however, relatively few studies exist in examining the efficacy of CBT in adolescent populations. To date, several proponents have advocated for the conceptual modification of adult-oriented CBT for adolescent populations, with one RCT and several case series attempting to illuminate the potential role of CBT in the treatment of adolescent BN (Lock, 2005; Schapman-Williams, Lock, & Courturier, 2006;

Schmidt et al., 2007). Such adaptations of CBT in adolescent populations typically emphasize the need to acknowledge normative cognitive and emotional immaturity among adolescents, resulting in greater age-appropriate psycho-education, greater flexibility in homework assignments, and parental involvement to assist in behavioral experiments and modified dietary practices (Lock, 2005).

Treatment findings to date point towards promising findings, suggesting that an adolescent-oriented self-help CBT program may be helpful in alleviating both binge eating and purging episodes (Schmidt et al., 2007). Furthermore, a study of older adolescents revealed that an online CBT intervention was effective in reducing both cognitive and behavioral BN symptomatology, demonstrating similar rates of symptom remission to those found in adult studies in adult BN populations (Pretorius et al., 2009). However, despite promising preliminary evidence, further controlled studies are warranted in further explicating the efficacy of CBT in adolescent presentations of BN.

Family-based treatment. FBT-BN borrows conceptually from the well-established FBT-AN and shares similar core theoretical tenets, taking account of symptomatic similarities including an overvaluation of weight and shape, elevated eating concerns, and a tendency to under-report symptom severity, thus centrally leveraging parental involvement. However, FBT-BN is somewhat distinct in light of the ego-dystonicity of BN behavioral symptoms, as the primary symptoms of binge eating and purging are almost universally experienced as distressing and contrary to one's aims. Thus, FBT-BN features a more collaborative stance between parents and the adolescent in collectively devising strategies to overcome the distressing behavioral features of BN (Le Grange & Lock, 2007).

To date, two large research trials have demonstrated promising results, in that FBT-BN appears efficacious in bringing about symptom remission which remains robust at both 6- and 12-month follow-up, (Le Grange & Lock, 2007) demonstrating similar treatment outcome to a modified guided self-help program of cognitive behavioral therapy (Schmidt et al., 2007).

Psychopharmacological treatment. To date only one trial has examined the pharmacological treatment of adolescent BN, demonstrating that adult doses of fluoxetine are not only well tolerated by adolescents, but may also bring about reductions in the frequency of binge and purge episodes, when administered alongside psychotherapy (Kotler, Devlin, Davies, & Walsh, 2003). Although this finding mirrors the findings of trials conducted in adult populations, further research is undoubtedly warranted in further expanding our understanding of the role of psychopharmacology in adolescent BN.

Binge Eating Disorder

Cognitive behavioral therapy. As with BN, CBT is currently the most well-established treatment for adult BED (Hay, 2013), prompting its adaptation for use in adolescent populations. CBT for BED is similar to the approach prescribed for

BN in its focus on normalizing eating patterns and improving distorted cognitions regarding eating, shape, and weight, with the added inclusion of a focus on enhancing acceptance of a larger-than-average body size, given the disorder's frequent overlap with obesity (e.g., Hudson, Hiripi, Pope, & Kessler, 2007). Adolescent-specific adaptations often include minimization of the abstract components of CBT (e.g., cognitive restructuring) coupled with an emphasis on providing concrete examples with personal relevance to teens; increased attention to adolescents' need for autonomy; and an enhanced focus on motivational techniques (Hilbert, Hartmann, Czaja, & Schoebi, 2013).

Several small trials have tested the efficacy of CBT for adolescent BED. Most recently, Debar, Wilson, Yarborough, Burns, and Oyler (2013) found that CBT out-performed a delayed treatment control condition in terms of binge abstinence and concomitant eating-, shape-, and weight-related concerns at post-treatment and 6-month follow-up. In Jones and colleagues' (2008) trial of Internet-delivered CBT for overweight teens, CBT led to a significant reduction in binge eating, BMI, z-BMI, and shape and weight concerns as compared to a waitlist control group.

Interpersonal psychotherapy. Interpersonal psychotherapy (IPT), which is considered a credible alternative to CBT for adult BED (Hay, 2013), assumes that binge eating results from deficits in interpersonal functioning (e.g., unresolved grief over the loss of a relationship, interpersonal role disputes) and subsequent experiences of negative affect. IPT's focus on improving relationship function for youth with binge eating may be especially relevant given the importance of peer relationships during adolescence, and evidence suggesting a strong link between interpersonally driven negative affect and loss binge eating in youth (Elliott, Tanofsky-Kraff, Shomaker, Columbo, & Wolkoff, 2010). Goals for treatment include elucidating connections between interpersonal triggers and subsequent binge eating, so that these patterns may be modified through the use of techniques such as social skills training and role negotiation. Data from a large, randomized controlled trial suggest that interpersonal psychotherapy significantly decreases the frequency of binge eating, and may curb weight gain among adolescent girls (Tanofsky-Kraff et al., 2014), and studies of cultural adaptations designed to enhance the suitability of the intervention for African American adolescents are underway (Cassidy, Sbrocco, & Tanofsky-Kraff, 2013).

Summary

Eating disorders remain a significant concern during adolescence, with an increasing prevalence alongside an ongoing resistance to conventional treatments. However, the relatively recent surge of treatments specifically oriented towards adolescents has positively impacted treatment outcomes in these populations. Furthermore, the delineation of factors that moderate and mediate treatment outcome (Le Grange et al., 2012) has further allowed for a more refined analysis and streamlining of the active components of treatment. What remains, however, is the notion that eating disorders during adolescence ought to be taken very seriously by those who encounter them.

Take-Home Points

- Eating disorders are serious psychiatric illnesses, which are associated with prolonged illness duration and marked medical complexities.
- Eating disorders most often have an onset during adolescence.
- Early intervention results in the most favorable treatment outcomes.
- High school personnel may detect early warning signs of eating disorders.
- A range of evidence-based treatments exists for adolescent eating disorders, and high school personnel should be familiar with various treatment approaches.

Resources

- Academy of Eating Disorders: www.aedweb.org
- National Association for Males with Eating Disorders: www.namedinc.org
- Families Empowered & Supporting Treatment for Eating Disorders: www.feast-ed.org

References

American Psychiatric Association (APA). (2013). *Diagnostic and statistical manual of mental disorders* (5th ed.) (DSM-5). Washington, DC: American Psychiatric Association.

Attia, E. (2010). Anorexia nervosa: Current status and future directions. *Annual Review of Medicine, 61*, 425–435.

Balestrieri, M., Oriani, M.G., Simoncini, A., & Bellantuono, C. (2013). Psychotropic drug treatment in anorexia nervosa. Search for differences in efficacy/tolerability between adolescent and mixed-age population. *European Eating Disorders Review, 21*, 361–373.

Brandenburg, B., Lesser, J., Mangham, D., & Crow, S. (2011). Psychopharmacological interventions for adolescents with eating disorders. *Adolescent Psychiatry, 1*, 277–285.

Bulik, C.M., Berkman, N.D., Brownley, K.A., Sedway, J.A., & Lohr, K.N. (2007). Anorexia nervosa treatment: A systematic review of randomized control trials. *International Journal of Eating Disorders, 40*, 310–320.

Cassidy, O., Sbrocco, T., & Tanofsky-Kraff, M. (2013). Utilizing non-traditional research designs to explore culture-specific risk factors for eating disorders in African-American adolescents. *Advances in Eating Disorders: Theory, Research and Practice, 38*, 965–977.

Couturier, J., Kimber, M., & Szatmari, P. (2013). Efficacy of family-based treatment for adolescents with eating disorders: A systematic review and meta-analysis. *International Journal of Eating Disorders, 46*, 3–11.

Dare, C., & Eisler, I. (2000). A multi-family group day program treatment programme for adolescent eating disorder. *European Eating Disorder Review, 8, 4–18.*

Debar, L.L., Wilson, G.T., Yarborough, B.J., Burns, B., & Oyler, B. (2013). Cognitive behavioral treatment for recurrent binge eating in adolescent girls: A pilot trial. *Cognitive and Behavioral Practice, 20*, 147–161.

Eddy, K.T., Dojer, D.J., Franko, D.L., Tahilani, K., Thomptson-Brenner, H., & Herzog, D.B. (2008). Diagnostic crossover in anorexia nervosa and bulimia nervosa: Implications for DSM-V. *American Journal of Psychiatry, 165*, 245–250.

Elliott, C.A., Tanofsky-Kraff, M., Shomaker, L.B., Columbo, K.M., & Wolkoff, L.E. (2010). An examination of the interpersonal model of loss of control eating in children and adolescents. *Behavior Research and Therapy, 48*, 424–428.

Fairburn, C.G. (2008). *Cognitive behavior therapy and eating disorders.* New York: Guilford Press.

Fisher, C.A., Hetrick, S.E., & Rushford. (2010). Family therapy for Anorexia Nervosa. The Cochrane collaboration. *The Cochrane Library, 6.*

Fitzpatrick, K.K., Moye, A., Hoste, R., Lock, J., & Le Grange, D. (2010). Adolescent focused psychotherapy for adolescents with anorexia nervosa. *Journal of Contemporary Psychotherapy, 40*, 31–39.

Goldschmidt, A.B., Jones, M., Manwaring, J.L., Luce, K.H., Osborne, M.I., Cunning, D., . . . Taylor, C.B. (2008). The clinical significance of loss of control over eating in overweight adolescents. *International Journal of Eating Disorders, 41*, 153–158.

Gowers, S., & Bryant-Waugh, R. (2004). Management of child and adolescent eating disorders: The current evidence base and future directions. *Journal of Child Psychology and Psychiatry, 45*, 63–83.

Gowers, S., Clark, A., Roberts, C., Griffiths, A., Edwards, V., Bryan, C., . . . Barrett, B. (2007). Clinical effectiveness of treatments for anorexia nervosa in young people: Randomised controlled trial. *The British Journal of Psychiatry, 191*, 427–435.

Grave, R.D., Calugi, S., Doll, H.A., & Fairburn, C.G. (2013). Enhanced cognitive behaviour therapy for adolescents with anorexia nervosa: An alternative to family therapy? *Behaviour, Research and Therapy, 51*, R9–R12.

Grilo, C.M. (2013). Why no cognitive body image feature such as overvaluation of shape/weight in binge eating disorder diagnosis? *International Journal of Eating Disorders, 46*, 208–211.

Hay, P. (2013). A systematic review of evidence for psychological treatments in eating disorders: 2005–2012. *International Journal of Eating Disorders, 46*, 462–469.

Hilbert, A., Hartmann, A.S., Czaja, J., & Schoebi, D. (2013). Natural course of preadolescent loss of control eating. *Journal of Abnormal Psychology, 122*, 684–693.

Hudson, J. I,. Hiripi, E., Pope, H.G., & Kessler, R.C. (2007). The prevalence and correlates of eating disorders in the National Comorbidity Survey replication. *Biological Psychiatry, 61*, 348–358.

Johnson, W.G., Rohan, K.J., & Kirk, A.A. (2002). Prevalence and correlates of binge eating in white and African American adolescents. *Eating Behaviors, 3*, 179–189.

Jones, M., Luce, K.H., Osborne, M.I., Taylor, K., Cunning, D., Celio-Doyle, A., . . . Taylor, C.B. (2008). Randomized controlled trial of an internet-facilitated intervention for reducing binge eating and overweight in adolescents. *Pediatrics, 121*, 453–462.

Kafantaris, V., Leigh, E., Hertz, S., Berest, A., Schebendach, J., Sterling, W. M, . . . Malhotra, A.K. (2011). A placebo controlled pilot study of adjunctive olanzapine for adolescents with anorexia nervosa. *Journal of Child and Adolescent Psychopharmacology, 21*, 207–212.

Keel, P.K., & Brown, T.A. (2010). Update on course and outcome in eating disorders. *International Journal of Eating Disorders, 43*, 195–204.

Kohn, M., & Golden, N.H. (2001). Eating disorders in children and adolescents: Epidemiology, diagnosis and treatment. *Paediatric Drugs, 3*, 91–99.

Kotler, L.A., Devlin, M.J., Davies, M., & Walsh, B.T. (2003). An open trials of fluoxetine for adolescents with bulimia nervosa. *Journal of Child and Adolescent Psychopharmacology, 13*, 329–335.

Lebow, J., Sim, L.A., Erwin, P.J., & Murad, M.H. (2013). The effect of atypical antipsychotic medication in individuals with anorexia nervosa: A systematic review and meta-analysis. *International Journal of Eating Disorders, 46,* 332–339.

Le Grange, D., & Eisler, I. (2009). Family interventions in adolescent anorexia nervosa. *Child and Adolescent Psychiatric Clinics of North America, 18,* 159–173.

Le Grange, D., & Lock, J. (2007). *Treating bulimia in adolescents: A family-based approach.* New York, NY: Guilford Press.

Le Grange, D., Lock, J., Agras, W.S., Bryson, S.W., Jo, B., & Kraemer, H.C. (2012). Mediators and moderators of remission in family-based treatment and adolescent focussed therapy for anorexia nervosa. *Behavior Research and Therapy, 50,* 85–92.

Lock, J. (2005). Adjusting cognitive behaviour therapy for adolescents with bulimia nervosa: Results of a case series. *American Journal of Psychotherapy, 59,* 267–281.

Lock, J., Couturier, J., & Agras, W.S. (2008). Costs of remission and recovery using family-based treatment for adolescent anorexia nervosa: A descriptive report. *Eating Disorders: The Journal of Treatment & Prevention, 4,* 322–330.

Lock, J., & Le Grange, D. (2013). *Treatment manual for anorexia nervosa: A family-based approach* (2nd ed.). New York, NY: Guilford Press.

Lock, J., Le Grange, D., Agras, W.S., Moye, A., Bryson, S., & Jo, B. (2010). Randomized control trial comparing family-based treatment with adolescent-focussed individual therapy for adolescents with anorexia nervosa. *Archives of General Psychiatry, 67,* 1025–1032.

Madden, S., Miskovic-Wheatley, J., Wallis, A., Kohn, M., Lock, J., Le Grange, D . . . Touyz, S. (2015). A randomized controlled trial of in-patient treatment for anorexia nervosa in medically unstable adolescents. *Psychological Medicine, 45,* 415–427.

Mond, J.M., Hay, P.J., Rodgers, B., Owen, C., & Beumont, P.J.V. (2005). Assessing quality of life in eating disorder patients. *Quality of Life Research, 14,* 171–178.

Murray, S.B., Loeb, K., & Le Grange, D. (2014). Indexing psychopathology throughout family-based treatment for adolescent anorexia nervosa: Are we on track? *Advances in Eating Disorders: Theory, Research and Practice, 2,* 93–96.

Neumark-Sztainer, D., Wall, M., Larson, N.I., Eisenberg, M.E., & Loth, K. (2011). Dieting and disordered eating behaviors from adolescence to young adulthood: Findings from a 10-year longitudinal study. *Journal of the American Dietetic Association, 111,* 1004–1011.

Pompili, M., Mancinelli, I., Girardi, P., Ruberto, A., & Tatarelli, R. (2004). Suicide in anorexia nervosa: A meta-analysis. *International Journal of Eating Disorders, 36,* 99–103.

Pretorius, N., Arcelus, J., Beecham J., Dawson, H., Doherty, F., Eisler, I., . . . Schmidt, U. (2009). Cognitive-behavioral therapy for adolescents with bulimic symptomatology: The acceptability and effectiveness of internet-based delivery. *Behavior Research and Therapy, 47,* 729–736.

Robin, A., Siegal, P., Koepke, T., Moye, A., & Tice, S. (1994). Family therapy versus individual therapy for adolescent females with anorexia nervosa. *Journal of Developmental and Behavioral Pediatrics, 15,* 111–116.

Robin, A., Siegal, P., Moye, A., Gilroy, M., Dennis, A., & Sikand, A. (1999). A controlled comparison of family versus individual therapy fort adolescents with anorexia nervosa. *Journal of the American Academy of Child and Adolescent Psychiatry, 38,* 1482–1489.

Rome, E.S., Ammermann, S., Rosen, D., Keller, R.J., Lock, J., Mammel, K.A., . . . Silber, T.J. (2003). Children and adolescent with eating disorders: The state of the art. *Paediatrics, 111,* e98–e108.

Schapman-Williams, A.M., Lock, J., & Courturier, J. (2006). Cognitive-behavioral therapy for adolescents with binge eating syndromes: A case series. *International Journal of Eating Disorders, 39,* 252–255.

Schmidt, U., Lee, S., Beecham, J., Perkins, S., Treasure, J., Yi, I., . . . Eisler, I. (2007). A randomized control trial of family therapy and cognitive behavior therapy guided self help care for adolescents with bulimia nervosa and related disorders. *American Journal of Psychiatry, 164*, 591–598.

Scholz, M., & Asen, E. (2001). Multiple family therapy with eating disordered adolescents: Concepts and preliminary results. *European Eating Disorders Review, 9*, 33–42.

Smink, F.R., van Hoeken, D., & Hoek, H.W. (2012). Epidemiology of eating disorder: Incidence, prevalence and mortality rates. *Current Psychiatry Reports, 14*, 406–414.

Steinhausen, H.C. (2002). The outcome of anorexia nervosa in the 20th Century. *American Journal of Psychiatry, 159*, 1284–1293.

Swanson, S.A., Crow, S.J., Le Grange, D., Swendson, J., & Merikangas, K.R. (2011). Prevalence and correlates of eating disorders in adolescents. *Archives of General Psychiatry, 68*, 714–723.

Tanofsky-Kraff, M., Shomaker, L.B., Wilfley, D.E., Young, J.F., Sbrocco, T., Stephens, M., . . . Yanovski, J.A. (2014). Targeted prevention of excess weight gain and eating disorders in high-risk adolescent girls: A randomized controlled trial. *American Journal of Clinical Nutrition, 100*, 1010–1018.

Treasure, J., & Russell, G. (2011). The case for early intervention in anorexia nervosa: Theoretical exploration or maintaining factors. *British Journal of Psychiatry, 199*, 5–7.

8

CHILDHOOD PHYSICAL HEALTH ISSUES IN THE SCHOOL CONTEXT

Paul C. McCabe and Katelyn Rose

Lorrie, age 16, has been diagnosed with type 1 diabetes since she was 7 years old. Lorrie has struggled to manage her health disorder while attempting to participate in activities typical for her same-age peers. She often finds herself too tired to participate in social activities and decides to stay home. As a result, Lorrie reports that she isn't dating and socializing with friends as much as she would like, and she has attributed her depressed mood and irritability to this. Her concentration and attention span vary widely, and on some days she is too distracted or fatigued to study and complete school work. Lorrie has struggled to maintain good grades even though she believes she is "pretty smart." She has developed vision problems secondary to her diabetes that also contribute to her fatigue and onset of headaches, despite corrective eyewear. Problems with excessive thirst and frequent bathroom trips for urination are noted in her teacher reports from previous school years. Lorrie manages her diabetes through regular blood sugar monitoring, at least 5–6 times a day, followed by insulin injections and medications as needed. She has found that maintaining consistent blood sugar and insulin levels has become much more challenging since the onset of puberty and menstruation. Lorrie is looking forward to living independently at university and developing an active social life, but has ongoing concerns about her ability to manage her diabetes on her own.

Winston has struggled with asthma most of his life. When he was younger, he suffered frequent bouts of croup and bronchiolitis brought on by RSV (respiratory syncytial virus). He often wheezed and complained of shortness of breath even after mild physical activity. At age 5, he suffered his first asthma attack while playing on the playground and was diagnosed with asthma. Now at age 8, Winston has learned to manage his asthma, but he reports that this isn't easy. He finds it harder to breathe, both indoors and outside of his apartment, and even light physical activity can bring on an attack. Winston complains that many adults in his family smoke in the apartment, making his breathing more labored. He loves to play basketball, but gets easily out of breath; because he needs to rest frequently, his friends no longer invite him to the courts. Winston tends to stay indoors and plays video games for many hours at a time. He needs to take medicine and inhaler treatments (corticosteroids) regularly at home as well as at school. Despite this ongoing treatment, Winston reports that on some days it is very difficult to regulate his breathing and this makes it challenging to concentrate on his school work. Some days he stays home from school because his breathing is too difficult. Winston is at-risk of failing 3rd grade due to excessive school absences. At his last doctor's visit, his pediatrician expressed concern about Winston's significant weight gain, which he believes may exacerbate his asthma symptoms. Winston expressed that he wishes to play basketball more with his friends and hopes that his breathing will improve so this will be possible.

Despite significant advances in medicine and preventative health care, pediatric health issues remain a consistent public health concern. Moreover, in the cases of some disorders, the prevalence rates are increasing despite advanced medical technologies. Childhood asthma has been diagnosed in 14% (1 in 7) of U.S. children under the age of 18, and many of these children continue to be diagnosed with asthma in adulthood (Bloom, Jones, & Freeman, 2013). Between 2001 and 2009, asthma rates rose almost 50% among African American children, and more than half of all children who had an asthma attack missed day(s) of school (Centers for Disease Control and Prevention, 2011). In the U.S., over 18,000 people younger than 20 years old are diagnosed with type 1 diabetes every year, and the prevalence rate is increasing in the United States, Canada, Australia, and Europe (Centers for Disease Control and Prevention, 2014; Lipman et al., 2013). One U.S. study found a 29% increase in type 1 diabetes in the past 20 years (Lipman et al., 2013).

Overall, there is a striking rise in the prevalence of chronic health conditions of childhood over the past few decades. One study found that chronic health conditions among children in the United States more than doubled from 12.8% in 1994 to 26.6% in 2006 (Van Cleave, Gortmaker, & Perrin, 2010). Asthma, obesity, and mental health disorders are among the conditions showing the greatest increase in the past three decades. Chronic health conditions make it more difficult for children to attend school and to concentrate when they do attend. For example, in 2008, school children in the United States missed 1.4 million days of school because of asthma (American Lung Association, 2010). School absences have consistently been associated with poorer academic performance, lower scores on standardized tests, and greater drop-out rates (Meng, Babey, & Wolstein, 2012).

Pediatric physical health conditions, such as asthma and diabetes, have a profound effect on a child's ability to effectively function in a school setting. School-age children afflicted with such issues are met with myriad physical, adaptive, cognitive, psychosocial, and behavioral difficulties. Modern medicine and improved treatment capabilities have helped many children survive what would once be fatal in the past, and therefore children are living and thriving with such medical conditions. However, parents, teachers, and caregivers often face the challenge of maintaining the health and well-being of children in their care. Within the school context, the impact of a student's disease, disorder, or impairment alters the educational environment and affects not only the child and those who help to manage the child's health issues, but all those who come into contact and interact with the child. At home, managing and caring for a child with chronic health difficulties can cause additional stress and tax resources as well as patience, which may further exacerbate symptoms and impact quality of care. A comprehensive approach to addressing physical health problems in children is best framed through examination of the social-ecological systems in which the child, family, school, health system, and social structures interact and impact the child's health (Shaw & McCabe, 2008).

Assessment and Identification

The child's first physical assessment and diagnosis is by a medical doctor or team. Young children visit their pediatricians regularly for well-child evaluations, where they receive preventive treatments (e.g., inoculations) and are screened for known risk factors of health disorders. The purpose of developmental assessments is to identify emerging or established medical disorders, or highlight risk factors or "red flags" for disorders that have not yet developed. In screening for known risk factors, problems will be discovered before they have time to fully develop (Edwards & Titman, 2010). Full physical examinations that monitor vision, hearing, blood pressure, vitamin deficiencies, and height and weight should be given annually to school-age children. Age-appropriate immunizations should also be administered. In addition, lifestyle habits, including diet, exercise, and sleep schedules should be closely observed by caregivers and reported to the family physician (Riley, Locke, & Skye, 2011).

Caregivers and school professionals have an important role in referring children to medical professionals if they suspect any abnormalities in a child's appearance, apparent health status, developmental and cognitive abilities, or behavior. Further medical assessment may be conducted based on the physical screening and recommendations of the medical team to confirm diagnoses and treatment options. To help with assessment and potential diagnosis, school performance can be used as developmental surveillance (Riley et al., 2011). In addition, school nurses play a valuable role in assessment of students as they possess the expertise to make informed decisions regarding student health care on a daily basis (Engelke, Guttu, Warren, & Swanson, 2008).

Effect on Academic Functioning

A major issue with regard to childhood health issues is the amount of time absent from school. Children suffering from health issues frequently miss school due to symptoms, doctor appointments, and effects from treatment (Shaw & McCabe, 2008). These absences unavoidably cause lapses in instructional time and learning, making it difficult for these children to catch up and remain on a grade-level academic trajectory. Due to frequent absences as well as pain, anxiety, and other symptomatology caused by illness, children with such health issues are at risk for poor academic outcomes (Engelke et al., 2008). When in school, children suffering from physical ailments may experience weakened cognitive abilities as well as a lack of motivation to complete school work. This decrease in ability and energy is often due to disease-related symptoms as well as various side effects from medication. Side effects from treatment regimens can greatly impact a child's executive functioning abilities, arousal, and new learning (Shaw & McCabe, 2008).

Dependent on the specific illness and treatment regime, a child may experience a range of symptoms and side effects that influence their ability to successfully function in school. Some medical conditions, specifically those that affect the central nervous system, such as epilepsy, are correlated with heightened rates of general or specific learning disabilities (Edwards & Titman, 2010). Treatment regimes that affect the central nervous system, such as treatment for certain types of cancer, can also result in learning disabilities that are often subtle and not easy to diagnose (Edwards & Titman, 2010). For example, treatments for childhood leukemia such as central nervous system prophylaxis and radiation therapy have been associated with cognitive deficits and learning problems post-treatment (McCabe, 2010). Other health conditions carry different symptoms that impact learning, and these symptoms may not initially be considered among the primary disease symptoms. For example, a child diagnosed with asthma may experience malaise or sleep loss and, when using beta-agonists, may face temporary fine-motor dysfunction. A child diagnosed with diabetes may experience acute hypo- or hyperglycemia, which affects attention, memory, learning, and processing speed (Shaw & McCabe, 2008).

At the school level, staff and health care providers, particularly school nurses, should partner with families and medical providers to ensure that students undergoing such health issues are afforded the same learning opportunities as typically developing children (Engelke et al., 2008). To do so, the full range of disease symptomatology, related effects, secondary conditions, and treatment side effects must be clearly communicated to all individuals who are working with those students. If a substantial amount of schooling has been missed due to a prolonged student absence, schools and families must work together to implement a transition plan that will accommodate a student's varied needs. A transition plan may include provisions for homebound instruction, flexible attendance, and differentiated teaching methods, as well as physical and social supports (Shaw & McCabe, 2008).

Evidence-based Interventions

Front-line interventions, such as reducing disruptions to the school day, ensuring that the educational environment is safe, and providing case management when needed, will help children to successfully manage their illnesses (Engelke et al., 2008). When in the classroom, teachers who teach children with special health needs are likely to be more successful when utilizing differentiated instruction and individually tailored learning strategies (Robinson & Summers, 2011). During this instruction, it is vital for teachers to take into account how the child's symptoms and treatment regime may affect their cognition and ability to learn (Robinson & Summers, 2011).

Another important primary intervention is the employment of a full-time, on-site school nurse. In terms of teacher perceptions of school nurse services, studies show that when there is a school nurse on-site there are fewer early releases due to illness, increased communication between school, family and the medical team, less teacher time spent on health problems, more time devoted to teaching, safer environments for students with chronic health problems, and increased use of the nurse as a personal resource for health and wellness information (Hill & Hollis, 2011). Dependent on the specifics of the illness or disease, more intensive interventions may be adopted. For example, model interventions for asthma would include avoiding known asthma triggers, maintaining a rescue inhaler with appropriate label at school, and creating a plan for staff to assist the student when using the rescue inhaler. Model interventions for diabetes may include decreasing episodes of hypoglycemia and hyperglycemia, as well as mandating that teachers and staff complete a diabetes management training (Engelke et al., 2008).

In terms of working directly with a child who has physical health issues in a school setting, all staff who come into contact with the child should have a fundamental understanding of the child's illness or disability (Kraft & Donoghue, 2010). School staff training should include information on the nature of the medical condition, related symptoms and side effects, and impact of the condition on the child's ability to function, focus, and participate in school. School staff who care for the child must be able to recognize signs and symptoms of impending medical problems as well as utilize appropriate techniques for feeding and handling. Staff should also be appropriately trained in the proper use and care of the child's adaptive equipment, if such equipment is needed (Kraft & Donoghue, 2010). To condense this important information for ease of use and reference, all children with a special health care needs should have a care plan which documents specific medical information, medication requirements and administration instructions, modifications needed in daily activities like diet or transportation, and emergency response information (Kraft & Donoghue, 2010).

Administering medication in schools can be a complex and risky task that may result in increased liability for schools and/or those handling the administration. School districts must have distinct and clear policies that comply with federal and state laws to support the safe administration of student medication. Within such policies, it is important to address physician authorization, parental consent, storage and dosage requirements, transport of medications, security and access issues, as well as training and supervision of school personnel who will administer any medication (Mazur-Mosiewicz, Pierson, & McIntosh, 2009). School team members, the student, the family, and medical professionals must collaborate on the delegation of medication to other parties (Mazur-Mosiewicz et al., 2009). Delegation of medication administration to others becomes particularly pertinent if the student leaves the school building for extracurricular activities, such as field trips or sporting events.

Psychosocial Effects

Effects of illness and treatment regimens coupled with time away from school can greatly hinder a child's ability to participate in school activities and may increase their risk for psychosocial difficulties. Long-term attendance problems due to illness may exacerbate already strained peer relationships and make it difficult to fully integrate within peer groups. Weiserbs and Gottlieb (2000) found that children with longstanding or permanent health issues or disabilities were at heightened risk for social isolation and stigma. Peer perception regarding a temporarily disabled same-age peer was found to be more favorable than peer perception of a peer with a permanent disability. In terms of befriending a peer with a permanently disabling condition, students were particularly apprehensive and fearful.

Because of the stigma associated with being sick or disabled, such children may internalize a feeling of difference or otherness, engendering a lower self-concept, and contributing to social skill deficits due to lack of social interactions (Verhoof, Maurice-Stam, Heymans, Evers, & Grootenhuis, 2014). As children with health conditions age, particularly those with chronic health issues, they often follow atypical development patterns and continue to adapt poorly to social situations (Verhoof et al., 2014). One study found that common psychosocial challenges of children with special health needs include a sense of not fitting in, vulnerability to other people's insensitivity, difficulty coping with fear and anxiety, and an atypical dependence on parents (Kratz, Uding, Trahms, Villareale, & Kieckhefer, 2009). The ongoing management and treatment of the physical issue can be hindered due to social, emotional, or behavioral challenges, given the frequent co-occurrence of these internalizing and externalizing social and emotional difficulties with physical ailment. There are helpful resources and websites for parents and teachers to explore the social and emotional consequences of chronic health difficulties, such as the website *HealthyChildren.org* created by the American Academy of Pediatrics (2014).

Issues of Culture

With respect to cultural differences and physical health issues among children, it is important that school professionals note the diverse and distinctive perceptions regarding illness among various cultural groups. Cultural variables, with particular regard to race, ethnicity, and socioeconomic status, play a major role in illness and health outcomes for children. There are many potential explanations for disparities in physical health functioning across cultures which may include differences in genetic predisposition and susceptibility to illness, divergent beliefs about health and wellness, lifestyle choices regarding diet and exercise, access to health care, environmental influences, and biases surrounding health care services (Clay, 2007).

In a study that examined Latino foster parents' health perceptions regarding their children's chronic medical conditions, it was found that the Latino parents surveyed had low levels of knowledge about chronic illness (Jee, Salter, Gonka, & Chin, 2014). They often believed that such health conditions held high spiritual significance and were determined by God. Many Latino families felt that alternative medicine and home remedies would be able to cure or help allay chronic illness. It was also found that the families had close familial ties and were highly nurturing to their children. Many of these families referenced the importance of extended kinship in caring for children who suffer from illness. Cultural attitudes, beliefs, and customs such as these should be viewed as valuable information at the school level. School teachers, social workers, psychologists and administrators would greatly benefit from such knowledge when interacting with caregivers because it will not only inform and prepare school staff in how to best approach child health concerns with families, but will build trust, cohesion, and foster further collaboration.

Due to the multitude of stressors afflicting children with debilitating health issues, a sensitive and devoted support network is essential. However, the challenges put on families of children with physical illnesses are also significant, making it difficult or impossible to manage independently of outside resources. As many health issues have a hereditary component, parents may also struggle with the same or similar incapacitating conditions, further exacerbating efforts to provide appropriate care for their child.

The Centers for Disease Control and Prevention and other researchers and health experts recommend the social-ecological model as a theoretical framework to help understand the nested factors that influence health and disease, including the impact of culture. This may include examination of individual risks, health, and behavior; nested within interpersonal contexts (i.e., family influence, peers, etc.); nested within institutions and organizations, communities, and societal systems, policies, and laws. As an example, the CDC has examined obesity with the social-ecological model to help understand obesity disparities, health behaviors, wellness, and treatment outcomes (Centers for Disease Control and Prevention, 2013).

For families of children with complex medical issues requiring intensive health care within the educational setting, studies show that families report a dearth of communication between primary care providers and educational specialists (Aruda, Kelly, & Newinsky, 2011). Parents of children with medically complex health issues also report that schools have difficulty in quickly adjusting services to accommodate medical crises after periods of relative stability (Aruda et al., 2011).

In light of these findings, it is of critical importance that a multidisciplinary team of family members, school professionals, and health care providers continuously maintain open lines of communication and coordinate to jointly manage care, with the end goal of improving child health outcomes and supporting the child's best quality of life.

As important as it is for a multi-disciplinary team to work together to care and plan for a child with health issues, it is expected that not all team members will have similar ideas about illness and health care. Social and cultural locations play a major role in one's conception of physical health issues and greatly influence all who attend to the affected child (Wright, Burrows, & Rich, 2012). School, government policy, and curriculum and intervention approaches convey meaning that significantly shapes the way children perceive and assess their health. Children begin to make sense of their condition and its implications through their interactions with others, the medical team, media, and cultural practices (Wright et al., 2012). As children with chronic illnesses grow older, they further develop a conceptualization of their disability and their identity, which for many incorporates acceptance and integration of the disability. These cognitive representations, or illness cognitions, directly influence their psychological health (Verhoof et al., 2014).

Tackling childhood physical health issues within a school context is a multi-faceted and challenging endeavor. There are many aspects to a child's health and well-being, and it is important that schools serve each child's individual needs appropriately. Education within a school setting, as opposed to home or hospital-based instruction, is particularly important for children with health issues as they will have the opportunity to experience successes among their peers, form friendships, and be distracted from their illness and treatments (Mukherjee, Lightfoot, & Sloper, 2000).

Take-Home Points

- The prevalence of childhood health disorders has risen in the past several decades, despite improvements in medical technologies.
- School professionals are increasingly faced with the multi-faceted challenge of care and management of children with physical health issues.
- Children with physical health issues are at risk for poor academic outcomes due to a high rate of school absence as well as inhibited cognitive abilities resulting from illness symptoms and treatment side effects.
- School-wide interventions to improve the safety and education of children with physical health issues should include the creation and implementation of in-school care plans, teacher utilization of differentiated instruction, school nurse employment, and staff training on specific special health needs within the student population.

- Psychosocial difficulties often plague children with physical health issues. Increased social isolation and stigma surrounding their disability can lead to low self-concept and poor interpersonal skills.
- Cultural issues play a major role in informing illness perceptions and health care decisions for children with physical health problems. In order to effectively collaborate with families to best serve a child with physical health issues, school professionals must work with families and communities to better understand the diverse cultural backgrounds of their students.

Resources

- American Diabetes Association: http://www.diabetes.org/
- Asthma and Allergy Foundation of America: http://www.aafa.org/
- American Academy of Pediatrics: http://www.aap.org
- Centers for Disease Control and Prevention: http://www.cdc.gov
- Healthy Child Care America: http://www.healthychildcare.org/
- National Resource Center for Health & Safety in Child Care and Early Education: http://www.nrckids.org
- Center for Parent Information & Resources: http://www.parentcenterhub.org/
- National Association of Pediatric Nurse Practitioners: http://www.napnap.org/

References

American Academy of Pediatrics. (2014). *Children with chronic illness: Dealing with emotional problems and depression.* Retrieved from http://www.healthychildren.org/English/health-issues/conditions/chronic/Pages/Children-with-Chronic-Illness-Dealing-with-Emotional-Problems-and-Depression.aspx

American Lung Association. (2010). *Trends in asthma morbidity and mortality.* Washington, DC: American Lung Association.

Aruda, M., Kelly, M., & Newinsky, K. (2011). Unmet needs of children with special health care needs in a specialized day school setting. *The Journal of School Nursing, 27*(3), 209–218. doi: 10.1177/1059840510391670

Bloom, B., Jones, L.I., & Freeman, G. (2013). Summary health statistics for U.S. children: National Health Interview Survey, 2012. National Center for Health Statistics. *VitalHealth Stat, 10*(258).

Centers for Disease Control and Prevention (CDC). (2011, May). Asthma in the US: Growing every year. *Vital Signs.* Retrieved from http://www.cdc.gov/vitalsigns/Asthma/?s_cid=vitalsigns_065

Centers for Disease Control and Prevention (CDC). (2013). Addressing obesity disparities: Social ecological model. Retrieved from http://www.cdc.gov/obesity/health_equity/addressingtheissue.html

Centers for Disease Control and Prevention (CDC). (2014). National diabetes statistics report: Estimates of diabetes and its burden in the United States, 2014. Atlanta, GA: U.S. Department of Health and Human Services.

Clay, D. L. (2007). Culturally competent interventions in schools for children with physical health problems. *Psychology in the Schools, 44*(4), 389–396. doi: 10.1002/pits.20230

Edwards, M., & Titman, P. (2010). *Promoting psychological well-being in children with acute and chronic illness.* London, UK & Philadelphia, PA: Jessica Kingsley Publishers.

Engelke, M., Guttu, M., Warren, M., & Swanson, M. (2008). School nurse case management for children with chronic illness: Health, academic, and quality of life outcomes. *The Journal of School Nursing, 24*(4), 205–214. doi: 10.1177/1059840508319929

Hill, N., & Hollis, M. (2011). Teacher time spent on student health issues and school nurse presence. *The Journal of School Nursing, 28*(3), 181–186. doi: 10.1177/1059840511429684

Jee, S., Salter, M., Gonka, J., & Chin, N. (2014). Latino foster parent health perceptions of chronic conditions: A qualitative exploration. *Journal of Child & Family Studies, 23*(2), 373–380. doi: 10.1007/s10826-013-9719-0

Kraft, C., & Donoghue, E. (2010). *Managing chronic health needs in child care and schools: A quick reference guide.* Elk Grove Village, Illinois: American Academy of Pediatrics.

Kratz, L., Uding, N., Trahms, C., Villareale, N., & Kieckhefer, G. (2009). Managing childhood chronic illness: Parent perspectives and implications for parent-provider relationships. *The Journal of Collaborative Family HealthCare, 27*(4), 303–313. doi: 10.1037/a0018114

Lipman, T.H., Levitt Katz, L.E., Ratcliffe, S.J., Murphy, K.M., Aguilar, A., Rezvani, I., . . . Suarez, E. (2013, January 22). Increasing incidence of type 1 diabetes in youth: Twenty years of the Philadelphia Pediatric Diabetes Registry. *Diabetes Care*, 1–7. doi: 10.2337/dc12–0767

Mazur-Mosiewicz, M., Pierson, E., & McIntosh, D. (2009). Legal issues in school health services and school psychology: Guidelines for the administration of medication. *Psychology in the Schools, 46*(9), 813–819. doi: 10.1002/pits.20421

McCabe, P.C. (2010). Cognitive effects of childhood leukemia treatments. In P.C. McCabe & S.R. Shaw (Eds.), *Pediatric disorders: Current topics and interventions for educators.* (pp. 61–70). Thousand Oaks, CA: Corwin Press.

Meng, Y., Babey, S.H., & Wolstein, J. (2012). Asthma-related school absenteeism and school concentration of low-income students in California. *Preventing Chronic Disease, 9*, 110312. doi: http://dx.doi.org/10.5888/pcd9.110312

Mukherjee, S., Lightfoot, J., & Sloper, P. (2000). The inclusion of pupils with a chronic health condition in mainstream school: What does it mean for teachers? *Educational Research, 42*(1), 59–72. doi: 10.1080/001318800363917

Riley, M., Locke, A., & Skye, E. (2011). Health maintenance in school-aged children: Part I. History, physical examination, screening, and immunizations. *American Family Physician, 83*(6), 683–688. Retrieved from http://www.aafp.org/journals/afp.html

Robinson, S., & Summers, K. (2011). An evaluation of the educational support for teachers who teach children with life-limiting illness in schools. *Pastoral Care in Education, 30*(3), 191–207. doi: 10.1080/02643944.2012.671341

Shaw, S.R., & McCabe, P.C. (2008). Hospital-to-school transition for children with chronic illness: Meeting the new challenges of an evolving health care system. *Psychology in the Schools, 45*(1), 74–87. doi: 10.1002/pits.20280

Van Cleave, J., Gortmaker, S.L., & Perrin, J.M. (2010). Dynamics of obesity and chronic health conditions among children and youth. *JAMA, 303*, 623–630. doi: 10.1001/jama.2010.104.

Verhoof, E.J.A., Maurice-Stam, H., Heymans, H.S.A., Evers, A.W.M., & Grootenhuis, M.A. (2014). Psychosocial well-being in young adults with chronic illness since childhood: The role of illness cognitions. *Child & Adolescent Psychiatry & Mental Health, 8*(1), 1–18. doi: 10.1186/1753-2000-8-12.

Weiserbs, B., & Gottlieb, J. (2000). The effect of perceived duration of physical disability on attitudes of school children toward friendship and helping. *The Journal of Psychology, 134*(3), 343–345. doi: 10.1080/00223980009600874

Wright, J., Burrows, L., & Rich, E. (2012). Health imperatives in primary schools across three countries: Intersections of class, culture and subjectivity. *Discourse: Studies in the Cultural Politics of Education, 33*(5), 673–691. doi: http://dx.doi.org/10.1080/01596306.2012.696500

9

ADOLESCENT SEXUALITY: CURRENT DIRECTIONS IN RESEARCH, HEALTH, AND RISK REDUCTION

Melanie J. Zimmer-Gembeck, Lucia F. O'Sullivan, Shawna Mastro, and Gillian Hewitt-Stubbs

Sexuality is often defined to include sexual behavior, the development of sexual preferences, the understanding of the self as a sexual being, sexual decision-making, and agency (Vasilenko, Lefkowitz, & Welsh, 2014). It also incorporates the understanding of others' sexual desires, and how to approach and manage intimacy with another person. Although sexual development and sexuality are founded in biology (Harden, 2014; Rodgers & Rowe, 1993), they also evolve from new life experiences that become more prevalent in adolescence, including the tendency to form close, dyadic relationships with peers of the same and other sex, and increased autonomy to spend more time with peers without the presence or supervision of parents or other adults (Impett & Tolman, 2006; Savin-Williams & Diamond, 2004; Zimmer-Gembeck, Ducat, & Collins, 2011; Zimmer-Gembeck, 2002). Thus, it is not surprising that all aspects of sexuality develop rapidly, expand with sexual expression and depth of experience during adolescence (and early adulthood), and become highly salient features of adolescents' and early adults' daily lives.

In this chapter, we provide a brief review of current research on adolescent sexuality, and focus primarily on sexual behavior, conceptions of the sexual self, and sexual health. We begin by describing challenges in the study of adolescent sexual behavior, as well as the theoretical frameworks most utilized by researchers, before briefly summarizing what is known from research about the onset and progression of behavior, and the correlates of early onset sexual behavior. We highlight similarities and differences between male and female adolescents, and consider the role of sociocultural background. We then discuss other aspects of sexuality, most prominently sexual self-perceptions and their role in sexual health and satisfaction. Finally, we summarize some recent research on school programs designed to assist youth with their sexual behavior decisions and/or positive sexual development.

The Study of Adolescent Sexuality

The predominant emphasis of research in the past four decades has been on the risks associated with adolescent sexual behavior. Many scholars have adopted a problem orientation and used Problem Behavior Theory (Jessor & Jessor, 1977) or Social Control Theory (Hirschi, 1969) to guide their research on adolescent sexuality (e.g., Capaldi, Crosby, & Stoolmiller, 1996; Tubman, Windle, & Windle, 1996). Others have had the primary aim of understanding the correlates of sexual risk behavior in order to gather information useful to risk reduction programs to improve public health. For example, in some studies, the aims have been to understand adolescent sexual planning and decision-making to guide the development of better interventions to assist adolescents to delay sexual intercourse, improve condom use, or limit their number of sexual partners (e.g., Sieving, McNeely, & Blum, 2000).

Another perspective on adolescent sexual behavior has been described in longitudinal studies that emphasize sexuality as part of normative development, as well as continuing to note the importance of individual dispositions and social environments in the development of sexual behavior patterns. In these investigations, researchers have emphasized the importance of the unfolding of biological processes. In what could be called a Biosocial Model, along with extensions of this model (Rodgers & Rowe, 1993), sexual activity, unlike other behaviors that can be risky, has been described as an activity almost every person will engage in by young adulthood and throughout life. Because of the normative biological and social-relational aspects of sexual behavior, researchers with this perspective have acknowledged the importance of biological factors, such as hormones and physical maturation, and social factors related to maturation, such as dating, that may promote the onset and patterns of sexual behavior during adolescence.

Overall, such a variety of views highlights the fact that adolescents can both take risks and be responsible, and sexuality development can be a correlate of other problems but also is an essential component in intimacy, pleasure, and closeness, including the refinement of skills in acquiring and maintaining positive relationships and support throughout adulthood (Siebenbruner, Zimmer-Gembeck, & Egeland, 2007; Willoughby et al., 2007). These perspectives highlight sexuality as an important developmental task of adolescence and advance a developmental research agenda focused on positive sexual health promotion (Boislard-Pepin & Zimmer-Gembeck, 2012; Diamond, 2003; O'Sullivan, Meyer-Bahlburg, & McKeague, 2006) rather than viewing this component of human life as aberrant or deviant in its earliest forms.

Sexual Behavior

Onset and progression. There are countless surveys that provide information about how many adolescents are engaging in a range of different sexual behaviors.

In fact, searching the literature can produce literally thousands of reports from the last half-century alone on sexual behavior. This can make consolidating this information complex and confusing. Nevertheless, the most recent of these studies provide up-to-date age-, gender-, and racial/ethnic-specific rates of vaginal intercourse and, increasingly, other forms of sexual behavior, such as oral sex. In the U.S. and other countries, there are also comprehensive and diverse longitudinal datasets that have been ideal for exploring individual differences in sexual behavior from the earliest years of adolescence into adulthood, and differences in patterns and progress in sexuality across these age periods (for reviews, see Dir, Coskunpinar, & Ciders, 2014; Zimmer-Gembeck & Helfand, 2008).

What do these studies tell us? First, they tell us about rates and progression of sexual behavior with increasing age. It is clear that the majority of young people residing in the U.S. (and in some other Western countries, such as Australia and Canada) have first sexual intercourse before leaving secondary school, with a first experience of vaginal intercourse most common at ages 16 or 17 years (Rotermann, 2012; Longmore, Manning, Giordano, & Rudolph, 2004; Zimmer-Gembeck, Ducat, & Boislard-Pepin, 2011). This average timing of first sexual intercourse is similar, but sometimes slightly later (e.g., at 17 rather than 16 years), among adolescents in Western European countries (Boyce et al., 2006; Skinner, Smith, Fenwick, Fyfe, & Hendriks, 2008). Overall, by about age 16–17, 50–70% of Western adolescents have experienced sexual intercourse, and 70–90% report first sexual intercourse by age 18 (for a review, see Zimmer-Gembeck, 2013). Sexual behavior rates can vary from study to study within a country, however. For example, surveys show that the percentage of adolescents who report first vaginal intercourse by the end of grade 8 can be as low as 10% to as high as almost 40%, where adolescents in economically disadvantaged urban environments typically report earlier initiation of intercourse than other adolescents (e.g., O'Donnell, Myint-U, O'Donnell, & Stueve, 2003; Santelli et al., 2004; Waller & Dubois, 2004).

Second, sexual surveys tell us about gender and racial/ethnic differences. In general, the gap in age of sexual activity initiation between boys and girls seems to be closing (Grunbaum et al., 2004). Nevertheless, a large minority of studies from the U.S. still report that males have their first experience of intercourse earlier than females (see Zimmer-Gembeck & Helfand, 2008). The variability in rates of sexual behavior is explained in part by jointly considering gender and race/ethnicity. When both are considered, the proportion of non-Hispanic Black study participants can often explain the gender difference, because Black males tend to report the earliest onset of vaginal intercourse when compared to all other groups, including Black females (O'Sullivan, Mantsun, Harris, & Brooks-Gunn, 2007). However, even among Black American adolescents, the gender gap seems to be narrowing (L'Engle & Jackson, 2008).

Third, recent surveys inform us about sexual behaviors other than intercourse. For example, some studies report that rates of oral sex among teenagers are similar to rates of vaginal intercourse (Malacad & Hess, 2010) and that, if it is initiated, the onset of oral sex occurs just months earlier than the time of first vaginal intercourse (O'Sullivan et al., 2007). Moreover, although the increasing rate of oral sex among adolescents has been a concern expressed by many parents and policymakers in recent years, oral sex among adolescents does not seem to be more prevalent today compared to rates reported before the new millennium (Maticka-Tyndale, 2008). It is important to note, however, that there has been a tendency to overlook some of the sexual activity among the 1% to 15% of adolescents who report same-sex attraction (Boyce et al., 2006; Savin-Williams & Diamond, 2004), but surveys show that most same-sex attracted youth do engage in heterosexual vaginal intercourse at some time during their teen years (Halpern, 2011). In addition, the tendency to focus on vaginal intercourse equates onset of a partnered sexual life as occurring at first intercourse, when in fact many adolescents report a range of sexual activities, such as breast and genital fondling, long before first intercourse occurs (O'Sullivan et al., 2007). Moreover, much of their early partnered sexual life is sporadic, with extended delays between occasions, and most sexual experiences occurring within the context of a steady relationship (Giordano, Manning, & Longmore, 2006).

Fourth and finally, as described above for oral sex, surveys tell us about historical and cohort changes in adolescent sexual behavior. When rates from the 1970s, 1980s, 1990s, and later are compared, it seems that adolescents are more likely to delay first intercourse until the later teen years compared to adolescents growing up in the 1970s or 1980s (Maticka-Tyndale, 2008). Furthermore, today's adolescents are more knowledgeable about safe-sex behaviors, and they are better able to carry out these safe behaviors (e.g., using condoms) than adolescents in previous decades, suggesting that they in many ways have a more positive sexual health record than their parents' and often their grandparents' generations. Other good news is that less than 10% of adolescents report vaginal intercourse without any contraception in some surveys, although the proportion of youth reporting inconsistent use of contraceptives is higher than 10% in other surveys (Boyce et al., 2006; Finer & Philbin, 2013; Wielandt, Boldsen, & Knudsen, 2002). Further good news is that teens seem to limit their number of sexual partners when they are sexually active, with most reporting a history of 1 or 2 partners (Lindberg, Jones, & Santelli, 2008). On the other hand, in many countries (e.g., the U.S., the U.K., and New Zealand) adolescents continue to have a higher than desired rate of unintended pregnancy. In addition, rates of sexually transmitted infections (STIs) are still alarmingly high among young people. For example, the U.S. Centers for Disease Control and Prevention find that youth 15–24 years account for almost half of new infections annually (Satterwhite et al., 2013). One in four sexually active women in this age range has an STI, such as chlamydia (Forhan et al., 2009).

The correlates of sexual debut. The evidence regarding the correlates of early (usually defined as age 15 or earlier) onset of first vaginal intercourse has been summarized in four comprehensive reviews (Goodson, Evans, & Edmundson, 1997;

Kirby, 2002; Kotchick, Shaffer, Forehand, & Miller, 2001; Zimmer-Gembeck & Helfand, 2008). In these reviews, many correlates of earlier first sexual activity are described, ranging from person factors, such as earlier pubertal onset and a tendency towards more problem behavior, to religious factors, such as lower church attendance, to parenting factors, such as less monitoring of adolescents' behavior (e.g., parents having less knowledge about adolescents' whereabouts, interests, and activities or being less likely to set a curfew). Being involved in dating earlier is also a strong correlate of earlier sexual behavior. Of this range of correlates, it is difficult to identify precisely which contributes most to early sexual initiation, especially when considering the added complexity of how these factors interact with and buffer each other (e.g., see Kincaid, Jones, Sterrett, & Mckee, 2012). For example, the correlates of sexual initiation are intercorrelated with each other, suggesting complex pathways to sexual intercourse. For example, family factors, such as living in a two-parent home and the levels of parental warmth, are rarely associated with adolescent sexual intercourse when factors like dating behavior, deviance in friends, or adolescent problem behavior are also considered. Such findings across the studies summarized in these reviews (e.g., Zimmer-Gembeck & Helfand, 2008) suggest that family factors are not directly implicated in the onset of adolescents' sexual behavior, but are indirectly important via their roles in establishing the types of friends that adolescents will have, the problem behaviors such as substance use that adolescents will experiment with, and adolescents' attitudes and aspirations. A further example is found within the association of pubertal development and earlier sexual debut, where the association is indirect via puberty's role in prompting the earlier establishment of dating relationships (Siebenbruner et al., 2007; Zimmer-Gembeck & Collins, 2008).

The Sexual Self

Much like adults, male and female adolescents' sexual experiences can involve a spectrum of feelings, reactions, and appraisals. Researchers note that adolescents' sexual experiences can be emotionally and physically satisfying but also caution that they can prompt significant negative emotional reactions, such as guilt, shame, anger, regret, and disappointment (Impett & Tolman, 2006; Smiler, 2013). Other research has found that high levels of positive desire, pleasure, and satisfaction characterize almost all sexual experiences among young people, even when an occasional sexual problem emerges (O'Sullivan & Majerovich, 2008). One adaptive outcome of sexual experimentation during adolescence seems to be emotional and cognitive growth, such as developing a firmer or more positive sense of what it means to be a sexual partner and producing heightened feelings of confidence in one's ability to manage sexual and other intimate interactions. For example, research has shown that a greater range of sexual experiences in late adolescence and early adulthood is associated with enhanced reflection about the self and relationships and is associated with greater esteem about one's sexual self, the body, efficacy in the sexual domain; all of these feelings of sexual esteem and efficacy have been associated with greater general well-being and life satisfaction in late adolescents and early adulthood (Horne & Zimmer-Gembeck, 2005; Zimmer-Gembeck et al., 2011). Overall, many adolescent sexuality researchers, health experts, and educators are coming to recognize that individual sexual attitudes, perceptions, and related cognitions are core to sexual health and that these sociosexual attitudes and perceptions can sometimes be associated with experiences with sex and intimate relationships (O'Sullivan & Brooks-Gunn, 2005; Zimmer-Gembeck et al., 2011). For example, a recent 4-year longitudinal study of adolescents elucidated a bidirectional relationship, whereby sexual self-concept became more positive over time in response to gains in sexual experience, but improvements in sexual self-concept also sparked increases in sexual behavior over time (Hensel, Fortenberry, O'Sullivan, & Orr, 2011; see also O'Sullivan & Brooks-Gunn, 2005).

Another part of the developmental task of sexuality in the second decade of life is to clarify one's sexual orientation. For a substantial minority of young people, defining one's own sexual attractions can take extra cognitive and emotional effort. Between 10 and 20% of youths endorse at least one measure of nonexclusive heterosexuality across studies (Igartua, Thombs, Burgos, & Montoro, 2009). Same-sex attractions and timing of sexual identity development often do not synchronize (Diamond & Savin-Williams, 2000), and there has been a recent but strong history of challenging efforts to pigeonhole sexual identity and attractions for sexual-minority youth (Diamond, 2003).

Recent Progress in Promoting Adolescent Sexual Development

Many programs exist to reduce adolescent sexual risk behavior, including delaying sex until a later, more appropriate time in one's development; limiting the number of sexual partners; reducing the frequency of sexual behavior; and using protection against pregnancy, HIV, and other STIs (for a review, see Gavin, Catalano, David-Ferdon, Gloppen, & Markham, 2010). Almost all of these programs have been implemented and evaluated in the U.S.; however, there are also programs and evaluations available from many other countries (e.g., Givaudan, Leenen, Van de Vijver, Poortinga, & Pick, 2008; Hanass-Hancock, 2014). In general, reviews of the evidence suggest that group-based, comprehensive risk-reduction programs and school-based, comprehensive contraceptive education programs (Bennett & Assefi, 2005; Kohler, Manhart, & Lafferty, 2008) have stronger and longer-lasting benefits than abstinence-only or abstinence-plus programs. Experts in pregnancy prevention point out that an exclusive emphasis on sexual abstinence does not appear to be effective for delaying the initiation of sex as it has had little effect on reducing patterns of any form of sexual behavior during adolescence, and may in fact be linked to higher rates of unprotected sex once onset has occurred (Kirby,

2008). Even more concerning, it may also be detrimental, with one study reporting higher rates of unprotected sex once onset has occurred (Kirby, 2008).

The more promising approaches—comprehensive risk-reduction and contraceptive education programs—have some common features, including the behaviors they hope to change and the content included in the programs. Risk-reduction programs aim to reduce behaviors associated with STI transmission and unintended pregnancy, such as reducing the number of different sexual partners reported by adolescents and the use of protection during all sexual activity, while still upholding abstinence as a better method of avoiding intended pregnancy and infections. Similarly, contraceptive education programs include messages about abstinence and provide information on birth control methods, like condoms and hormonal methods, to prevent STIs and unintended pregnancy. For example, one school-based program, Safer Choices, focuses on delaying the initiation of sex, reducing the frequency of unprotected sexual intercourse, reducing the number of unprotected sexual partners, increasing condom use consistency, and increasing contraceptive use (Kirby et al., 2004; see also Kirby, Baumler, & Coyle, 2011). This program has five components of staff development, peer resources, school environment changes, parent education, and linking schools with community agencies. This large and intensive program has shown positive effects, albeit generally fairly small effects, on some of the targeted sexual risk behaviors in every group studied, including boys and girls, and in every sociocultural group. In another program evaluation of It's Your Game: Keep It Real, a program designed for grade 7 students to reduce pregnancy and HIV/STI rates, initiation of sex was reduced in the intervention group (n = 558) compared to a comparison group (n = 349; Tortolero et al., 2010). About 23% of the intervention group initiated sex by grade 9, whereas the rate was significantly higher at 30% in the comparison groups (see also Markham et al., 2012).

Many contemporary approaches in sexual risk avoidance focus on providing general skills that should serve adolescents when they need to avoid risk behavior across many domains. Although more research is needed to understand exactly what core beliefs and skills help young people, general positive youth development programs, which focus on a range of skills, such as promoting prosocial behavior, decision-making, and emotional competence, seem to be most promising as a sexual risk-reduction program (Gavin et al., 2010). A new direction in intervention is the use of technology to provide information to youth about sexual health or to provide a resource for youth to gain access to services. In general, in a recent review of 10 evaluations of programs using digital media (Guse et al., 2012), two of the programs were effective in delaying onset of sexual intercourse, but most have not shown this high level of effectiveness. However, multiple other interventions that were included in this review reported increased adolescent knowledge about sexual health and protective behaviors, or increased feelings of efficacy to engage in protective sexual health behaviors, following participation in their programs.

Conclusion

Recent theoretical frameworks that consider adolescent sexuality as normative and developmentally appropriate have fostered a greater understanding of sexuality and sexual well-being in young people, moving beyond risk behavior alone to include self-perceptions and feelings of pleasure, esteem, and intimacy that were once overlooked in this age group. This holistic approach can help reframe research and policy to better evaluate the antecedents and consequences of adolescent sexual behavior, in terms of both physical and mental health. Although useful to consider, correlates of early debut and other risk behavior on their own do not explain how and why risk behavior occurs. More likely, consideration of such factors with greater scope and complexity, such as how interpersonal skills, family factors, social environment, and pubertal onset interact provide a richer understanding of the circumstances in which risk behavior occurs. Similarly, intervention strategies with more scope—ones that emphasize and enhance interpersonal skills necessary to navigate sexual and romantic relationships, as well as provide factual information about pregnancy, STIs, contraception, and consent—are better at equipping adolescents with the tools to make sexually safe choices. It is within these safe choices that adolescents can experience the positive sexual development that is integral to their sexual and overall well-being and that, in addition, leaves them better prepared for future intimate relationships.

Take-Home Points

- Sexuality is a normative developmental task of adolescence, requiring a balanced focus on the risky aspects of sexual behavior as well as sexual health, well-being, and pleasure.
- The majority of young people in Western countries engage in some form of sexual behavior by age 17 to 18 years, but this varies with gender, ethnicity, economic status, family relationships, pubertal timing, and dating behavior.
- Young people today practice safe sex behaviors at levels at or better than generations before, but in many countries they still have concerning rates of sexual transmitted infections and unintended pregnancy.
- The best evidence suggests that general skills-based programs, which include risk-reduction and contraceptive information, provide the information, and the interpersonal, emotional, and decision-making skills that equip adolescents to more safely negotiate sexual relationships and experiences.

References

Bennett, S.E., & Assefi, N.P. (2005). School-based teenage pregnancy prevention programs: A systematic review of randomized controlled trials. *Journal of Adolescent Health*, *36*, 72–81.

Boislard-Pepin, M.A., & Zimmer-Gembeck, M.J. (2012). Adolescent sexual behavior: Current knowledge, challenges and implications for research and policy. In N.E. Peterson & W. Campbell (Eds.), *Handbook on sexuality: Perspective, issues, and role in society* (pp. 153–168). New York: NOVA Science Publishers.

Boyce, W., Doherty-Poirier, M., MacKinnon, D., Fortin, C., Saab, H., King, M., & Gallupe, O. (2006). Sexual health of Canadian youth: Findings from the Canadian Youth, Sexual Health and HIV-AIDS Study. *The Canadian Journal of Human Sexuality, 15*, 59–68.

Capaldi, D.M., Crosby, L., & Stoolmiller, M. (1996). Predicting the timing of first sexual intercourse for at-risk adolescent males. *Child Development, 67*, 344–359.

Diamond, L.M. (2003). Love matters: Romantic relationships among sexual-minority adolescents. In P. Florsheim (Ed.), *Adolescent romantic relations and sexual behavior: Theory, research, and practical implications* (pp. 85–107). Mahwah, NJ: Erlbaum.

Diamond, L.M., & Savin-Williams, R.C. (2000). Explaining diversity in the development of same-sex sexuality among young women. *Journal of Social Issues, 56*, 297–313.

Dir, A L., Coskunpinar, A., & Ciders, M.A. (2014). A meta-analytic review of the relationship between adolescent risky sexual behavior and impulsivity across gender, age, and race. *Clinical Psychology Review, 343*, 551–562.

Finer, L.B., & Philbin, J.M. (2013). Sexual initiation, contraceptive use, and pregnancy among young adolescents. *Pediatrics, 131*, 886–891.

Forhan, S.E., Gottlieb, S.L., Sternberg, M.R., Xu, F., Datta, S.D., McQuillan, G.M., . . . Markowitz, L.E. (2009). Prevalence of sexually transmitted infections among female adolescents aged 14 to 19 in the United States. *Pediatrics, 124*, 1505–1512.

Gavin, L.E., Catalano, R.F., David-Ferdon, C., Gloppen, K.M., & Markham, C.M. (2010). A review of positive youth development programs that promote adolescent sexual and reproductive health. *Journal of Adolescent Health, 46*, S75–S91.

Giordano, P.C., Manning, W.D., & Longmore, M.A. (2006). Adolescent romantic relationships: An emerging portrait of their nature and developmental significance. In A.C. Crouter & A. Booth (Eds.), *Romance and sex in adolescence and emerging adulthood: Risks and opportunities* (pp. 127–150). Mahwah, NJ: Erlbaum.

Givaudan, M., Leenen, I., Van de Vijver, F.J.R., Poortinga, Y.H., & Pick, S. (2008). Longitudinal study of a school based HIV/AIDS early prevention program for Mexican adolescents. *Psychology, Health & Medicine, 13*, 98–110.

Goodson, P., Evans, A., & Edmundson, E. (1997). Female adolescents and onset of sexual intercourse: A theory-based review of research from 1984–1994. *Journal of Adolescent Health, 21*, 147–156.

Grunbaum, J.A., Kann, L., Kinchen, S., Ross, J., Hawkins, J., Lowry, R., Harris, W.A., Mcmanus, T., Chyen, D., & Collins, J. (2004). Youth risk behavior surveillance—United States, 2004. *Morbidity and Mortality Weekly, 53*, 1–96.

Guse, K., Levine, D., Martins, S., Lira, A., Gaarde, J., Westmorland, W., & Gilliam, M. (2012). Interventions using new digital media to improve adolescent sexual health: A systematic review. *Journal of Adolescent Health, 51*, 535–543.

Halpern, C.T. (2011). Same-sex attraction and health disparities: Do sexual minority youth really need something different for healthy development? *Journal of Adolescent Health, 48*, 5–6.

Hanass-Hancock, J. (2014). Tangible skill building and HIV youth prevention intervention in rural South Africa. *African Journal of AIDS Research, 13*, 229–235.

Harden, K.P. (2014). A sex-positive framework for research on adolescent sexuality. *Perspectives on Psychological Science, 9*, 455–469.

Hensel, D., Fortenberry, D., O'Sullivan, L., & Orr, D. (2011). The developmental association of sexual self-concept with sexual behavior among adolescent women. *Journal of Adolescence, 84*, 675–684.

Hirschi, T. (1969). *Causes of delinquency*. Berkeley: University of California Press.

Horne, S., & Zimmer-Gembeck, M.J. (2005). Female sexual subjectivity and well-being: Comparing late adolescents with different sexual experiences. *Sexuality Research & Social Policy, 2*, 25–40.

Igartua, K., Thombs, B.D., Burgos, G., & Montoro, R. (2009). Concordance and discrepancy in sexual identity, attraction, and behavior among adolescents. *Journal of Adolescent Health, 45*, 602–608.

Impett, E.A., & Tolman, D.L. (2006). Late adolescent girls' sexual experiences and sexual satisfaction. *Journal of Adolescent Research, 21*, 628–646.

Jessor, S.L., & Jessor, R. (1977). *Problem behavior and psychosocial development: A longitudinal study of youth*. New York: Academic Press.

Kincaid, C., Jones, D.J., Sterrett, E., & McKee, L. (2012). A review of parenting and adolescent sexual behavior: The moderating role of gender. *Clinical Psychology Review, 32*, 177–188.

Kirby, D. (2002). Antecedents of adolescent initiation of sex, contraceptive use, and pregnancy. *American Journal of Health Behavior, 26*, 473–485.

Kirby, D.B. (2008). The impact of abstinence and comprehensive sex and STD/HIV education programs on adolescent sexual behavior. *Sexuality Research & Social Policy, 5*, 18–27.

Kirby, D.B., Baumler, E., & Coyle, K.K. (2011). The impact of 'Safer Choices' on condom use and contraceptive use among sexually experienced students at baseline. *Unpublished manuscript*.

Kirby, D.B., Baumler, E., Coyle, K.K., Basen-Engquist, K., Parcel, G.S., Harrist, R., & Banspach, S.W. (2004). The "Safer Choices" intervention: Its impact on the sexual behaviors of different subgroups of high school students. *Journal of Adolescent Health, 35*, 442–452.

Kohler, P.K., Manhart, L.E., & Lafferty, W.E. (2008). Abstinence-only and comprehensive sex education and the initiation of sexual activity and teen pregnancy. *Journal of Adolescent Health, 42*, 344–351.

Kotchick, B.A., Shaffer, A., Forehand, R. & Miller, K.S. (2001). Adolescent sexual risk behavior: A multi-system perspective. *Clinical Psychology Review, 21*, 493–519.

L'Engle, K.L., & Jackson, C. (2008). Socialization influences on early adolescents' cognitive susceptibility and transition to intercourse. *Journal of Research on Adolescence, 18*, 353–378.

Lindberg, L.D., Jones, R., & Santelli, J.S. (2008). Noncoital sexual activities among adolescents. *Journal of Adolescent Health, 43*, 231–238.

Longmore, M.A., Manning, W.D., Giordano, P.C., & Rudolph, J.L. (2004). Self-esteem, depressive symptoms, and adolescents' sexual onset. *Social Psychology Quarterly, 67*, 279–295.

Malacad, B.L., & Hess, G.C. (2010). Oral sex: Behaviours and feelings of Canadian young women and implications for sex education. *The European Journal of Contraception and Reproductive Health Care, 15*, 177–185.

Markham, C.M., Tortolero, S.R., Peskin, M.F., Shegog, R., Thiel, M., Baumler, E.R., . . . & Robin, L. (2012). Sexual risk avoidance and sexual risk reduction interventions for middle school youth: A randomized controlled trial. *Journal of Adolescent Health, 50*, 279–288.

Maticka-Tyndale, E. (2008). Sexuality and sexual health of Canadian adolescents: Yesterday, today and tomorrow. *The Canadian Journal of Human Sexuality*, *17*, 85–95.

O'Donnell, L., Myint-U, A., O'Donnell, C.R., & Stueve, A. (2003). Long-term influence of sexual norms and attitudes on timing of sexual initiation among urban minority youth. *Journal of School Health*, *73*, 68–75.

O'Sullivan, L.F., & Brooks-Gunn, J. (2005). The timing of changes in girls' sexual cognitions and behaviors in early adolescence: A prospective, cohort study. *Journal of Adolescent Health*, *37*, 211–219.

O'Sullivan, L.F., & Majerovich, J. (2008). Difficulties with sexual functioning in a sample of male and female late adolescent and young adult university students. *The Canadian Journal of Human Sexuality*, *17*, 109–121.

O'Sullivan, L.F., Mantsun, M., Harris, K.M., & Brooks-Gunn, J. (2007). I wanna hold your hand: The progression of social, romantic and sexual events in adolescent relationships. *Perspectives on Sexual and Reproductive Health*, *39*, 100–107.

O'Sullivan, L.F., Meyer-Bahlburg, H.F.L., & McKeague, I.W. (2006). The development of the sexual self-concept inventory for early adolescent girls. *Psychology of Women Quarterly*, *30*, 139–149.

Rodgers, J.L., & Rowe, D.C. (1993). Social contagion and adolescent sexual behavior: A developmental EMOSA model. *Psychological Review*, *100*, 479–510.

Rotermann, M. (2012). Sexual behaviour and condom use of 15- to 24-year-olds in 2003 and 2009/2010. *Health Reports*, *23*, 1–5.

Santelli, J. S, Kaiser, J., Hirsch, L., Radosh, A., Simkin, L., & Middlestadt, S. (2004). Initiation of sexual intercourse among middle school adolescents: The influence of psychosocial factors. *Journal of Adolescent Health*, *34*, 200–208.

Satterwhite, C.L., Torrone, E., Meites, E., Dunne, E.F., Mahajan, R., Ocfemia, M.C., . . . Weinstock, H. (2013). Sexually transmitted infections among US women and men: Prevalence and incidence estimates, 2008. *Sexually Transmiteed Diseases*, *40*, 187–193.

Savin-Williams, R.C., & Diamond, L.M. (2004). Sex. In L. Steinberg (Ed.), *Handbook of adolescent psychology* (pp. 189–225). Mahwah, NJ: Wiley.

Siebenbruner, J., Zimmer-Gembeck, M.J., & Egeland, B. (2007). Sexual partners and contraceptive use: A 16-year prospective study predicting abstinence and risk behavior. *Journal of Research on Adolescence*, *17*, 179–206.

Sieving, R.E., McNeely, C.S., & Blum, R.W. (2000). Maternal expectations, mother-child connectedness, and adolescent sexual debut. *Archives of Pediatrics & Adolescent Medicine*, *154*, 809–816.

Skinner, S.R., Smith, J., Fenwick, J., Fyfe, S., & Hendriks, J. (2008). Perceptions and experiences of first sexual intercourse in Australian adolescent females. *Journal of Adolescent Health*, *43*, 593–599.

Smiler, A.P. (2013). *Challenging Casanova: Beyond the stereotype of the promiscuous young male*. San Francisco, CA: Jossey-Bass.

Tortolero, S.R., Markham, C.M., Peskin, M.F., Shegog, R., Addy, R.C., Escobar-Chaves, S.L., & Baumler, E.R. (2010). It's Your Game: Keep It Real: Delaying sexual behavior with an effective middle school program. *Journal of Adolescent Health*, *46*, 169–179.

Tubman, J.G., Windle, M., & Windle, R.C. (1996). Cumulative sexual intercourse patterns among middle adolescents: Problem behavior precursors and concurrent health risk behaviors. *Journal of Adolescent Health*, *18*, 182–191.

Vasilenko, S.A., Lefkowitz, E.S., & Welsh, D.P. (2014). Healthy sex and sexual health: New directions for studying outcomes of sexual health. In E.S. Lefkowitz & S.A. Vasilenko

(Eds.), Positive and negative outcomes of sexual behaviors. *New Directions for Child and Adolescent Development, 144*, 3–19.

Waller, E.M., & Dubois, D.L. (2004). Investigation of stressful experiences, self-evaluations, and self-standards as predictors of sexual activity during early adolescence. *Journal of Early Adolescence, 24*, 431–459.

Wielandt, H., Boldsen, J., & Knudsen, L.B. (2002). The prevalent use of contraception among teenagers in Denmark and the corresponding low pregnancy rate. *Journal of Biosocial Science, 34*, 1–11.

Willoughby, T., Chalmers, H., Busseri, M.A., Bosacki, S., Dupont, D., Marini, Z., . . . Woloshyn, V. (2007). Adolescent non-involvement in multiple risk behaviors: An indicator of successful development? *Applied Development Science, 11*, 89–103.

Zimmer-Gembeck, M.J. (2002). The development of romantic relationships and adaptations in the system of peer relationships. *Journal of Adolescent Health, 31*, 216–225.

Zimmer-Gembeck, M.J. (2013). Young females' sexual-efficacy: Associations with personal autonomy and the couple relationship. *Sexual Health*. doi: 10.1071/SH12139

Zimmer-Gembeck, M.J., & Collins, W.A. (2008). Biological sex, appearance, alcohol use and dating as correlates of sexual partner accumulation from ages 16 to 26, *Journal of Adolescent Health, 42*, 564–572.

Zimmer-Gembeck, M.J., Ducat, W.H., & Boislard-Pepin, M.A. (2011). A prospective study of young females' sexual subjectivity: *Associations with age, sexual behavior, and dating. Archives of Sexual Behavior, 40*, 927–938.

Zimmer-Gembeck, M. J., Ducat, W., & Collins, W.A. (2011). Autonomy development during adolescence. In B.B. Brown & M. Prinstein (Eds.), *Encyclopedia of adolescence* (pp. 66–76). New York: Academic Press.

Zimmer-Gembeck, M.J., & French, J. (in press). Associations of sexual subjectivity with global and sexual well-being: A new measure for young males and comparison to females, *Archives of Sexual Behavior*. doi: 10.1007/s10508-014-0387-y

Zimmer-Gembeck, M.J., & Helfand, M. (2008). Ten years of longitudinal research on U.S. adolescent sexual behavior: The evidence for multiple pathways to sexual intercourse, and the importance of age, gender and ethnic background, *Developmental Review, 28*, 153–224.

10

MENTAL HEALTH CONCERNS AMONG LGBTQ YOUTH IN SCHOOLS

V. Paul Poteat, Ian Rivers, and Jillian R. Scheer

Over the past decade, a major focus and goal among researchers, practitioners, and policy makers working with sexual minority youth (e.g., lesbian, gay, bisexual, transgender, and queer or questioning youth; LGBTQ) has been to promote safer and more welcoming schools for this population. This focus has been driven by many factors, including the consistent finding that many LGBTQ youth experience homophobic harassment at school from peers and adults (Grossman & D'Augelli, 2006; Rivers, 2001; Russell, Everett, Rosario, & Birkett, 2014). Further, LGBTQ youth face pronounced disparities across many health and academic outcomes. For instance, LGBTQ youth report greater anxiety, depression, traumatic stress, truancy, poorer grades, less school belonging and safety, and less intent to graduate than heterosexual youth (Birkett, Russell, & Corliss, 2014; Coker, Austin, & Schuster, 2010; Poteat, Mereish, DiGiovanni, & Koenig, 2011). These sexual orientation-based disparities have been tied to the higher rates of victimization that LGBTQ youth experience compared to heterosexual youth. Because schools are one of the primary contexts in which children and adolescents spend most of their time, addressing the experiences of LGBTQ youth in this setting is critical to promoting their health and well-being.

Educators, psychologists, and other school professionals all have key roles in working with LGBTQ youth at school. To provide the most effective support and services, it is important to understand the experiences and needs of LGBTQ youth; further, it is essential to know what resources and practices are most effective in countering the discrimination and barriers faced by these youth and that promote their resilience. In this chapter, we first consider frameworks for understanding the experiences of LGBTQ youth in the school ecology and for explaining how disparities arise. Second, we focus on bullying and discrimination as major factors contributing to mental health concerns among LGBTQ youth.

Third, we discuss factors, resources, and policies at multiple levels that can promote resilience among LGBTQ youth. Finally, we note how research and interventions could expand in ways that could lead to even stronger efforts to ensure the long-term well-being and resilience of LGBTQ youth.

Developmental and Health Disparity Models Relevant to LGBTQ Youth in Schools

We rely on two theoretical models to frame our review of health concerns among LGBTQ youth in schools. The first model is the bioecological model (Bronfenbrenner & Morris, 2006). This model provides a framework for situating LGBTQ youth within the broader school context and for positioning the multiple factors that affect their experiences and their subsequent health. Based on this model, LGBTQ youth are situated within social systems, some of which are immediate and proximal to them (e.g., families, schools) and others that are more distal (e.g., the broader school district or community, society at large). Experiences within each of these social systems can overlap with one another (e.g., the effects of family rejection or support can affect LGBTQ youths' learning experiences at school); however, for the purpose of this chapter, we focus on the school context. In addition, factors at various levels, ranging from individual characteristics to interpersonal experiences to institutional policies, can shape the experiences of LGBTQ youth in schools. Although most of the extant work on LGBTQ youth has focused on individual or interpersonal factors, emerging research has begun to consider how more distal factors such as school policies may affect LGBTQ youths' experiences. This model thus provides a useful framework for cataloging the many factors that underlie LGBTQ youths' experiences at school and how they are interrelated.

The second model we rely upon is the minority stress model (Meyer, 2003). This model outlines the various pathways through which multiple factors lead to the health disparities documented among the LGBTQ population. In this way, the minority stress model complements the bioecological model by helping to understand how proximal and distal factors across multiple contexts interact with one another to either magnify or attenuate resulting health risks among the LGBTQ youth population. Minority stress theory postulates that individuals in marginalized positions in society face unique stressors connected to their marginalized identity; these stressors are in addition to other general life stressors and can be proximal or distal in nature. Distal stressors are external to the individual, such as discrimination (e.g., LGBTQ students may be assaulted by other students or excluded from peer groups) or social policies (e.g., school policies that prohibit discussion of LGBTQ issues in the classroom). Proximal stressors refer to internal psychological processes, such as internalized homophobia (e.g., an LGBTQ youth's internalization of negative societal beliefs that denigrate non-heterosexual identities) or heightened vigilance or rejection sensitivity on account of sexual orientation. The minority stress model argues that these unique stressors partly explain why LGBTQ individuals experience greater health risks than heterosexual individuals. Furthermore, the model proposes that factors can either exacerbate or attenuate the extent to which these stressors elevate risks for LGBTQ individuals. We highlight several of these factors later in the chapter.

School Bullying and Discrimination Against LGBTQ Youth

School-based discrimination experiences are a primary contributor to mental health concerns among LGBTQ youth. Several terms have been used to describe such discriminatory acts in a broad sense, such as bias-, stigma-, or identity-based bullying or harassment (e.g., homophobic bullying or harassment). Essentially, these various terms are meant to describe and capture acts of aggression directed toward someone based on that person's actual or assumed marginalized social identity (e.g., for identifying as or being perceived to be LGBTQ). The bullying of LGBTQ youth can take many forms. It can be physical (e.g. hitting, kicking, or punching), verbal (e.g. name-calling, use of homophobic epithets), or social (e.g. being ignored or excluded from the group).

Historic and Recent Trends of Homophobic Harassment

Exact prevalence rates of homophobic harassment of LGBTQ youth remain difficult to discern and vary across studies, partly because there are few representative population-based datasets that have assessed for homophobic harassment or that have collected information on youths' sexual orientation identity. Also, among those studies that have assessed for homophobic harassment, there has been variability in how it has been measured, with some studies including only overt or extreme indices, while others have included a range of behaviors. Nevertheless, some general trends are evident from data collected over the past two decades.

Early research on homophobic harassment among LGBTQ youth was primarily retrospective with some concurrent reports. In the late 1980s to early 1990s, reported rates of victimization varied widely across the U.S. and the U.K., two countries in which data were most consistently collected. These rates ranged from 12% to 59% (Gross, Aurand, & Adessa, 1988; Pilkington & D'Augelli, 1995), though a larger review of data from this time period generally estimated that 33% to 49% of LGB individuals were bullied at school (Berrill, 1992). Similar trends of homophobic harassment have been documented in the U.K. Ellis and High (2004) noted that there had been an increase in reports of bullying against LGB youth: Youth in 2001 were four times more likely to report feeling isolated at school than those in 1984. They were almost five times more likely to experience verbal abuse, seven times more likely to say they had been teased, three times more likely to be physically assaulted, five times more likely to be excluded from social gatherings by peers, and nine times more likely to feel "pressured to conform." Although explanations for these trends have been unable to be directly tested, it is possible that they might be tied to several contributing factors, such as the greater number of youth who now come out during adolescence, greater awareness of bullying behavior, greater comfort in disclosing such information, or backlash against LGBTQ youth even as advances are being made in other areas (e.g., anti-bullying policies).

In more recent periods, the organization GLSEN (Gay, Lesbian and Straight Education Network) has tracked school-based bullying of LGBTQ youth over time. In their 2011–2012 report (Kosciw, Greytak, Bartkiewicz, Boesen, & Palmer, 2012), GLSEN found that 63.5% of the 8,584 LGBTQ youth they surveyed said they felt unsafe at school because of their sexual orientation and 43.9% because of their gender expression. Of those who felt unsafe, 81.9% reported having been called names or threatened in the last 12 months because of their sexual orientation, and 63.9% because of their gender expression. The U.K.-based group Stonewall surveyed 1,145 lesbian, gay, and bisexual (LGB) students enrolled in secondary schools and colleges in 2007 to assess their experiences of homophobic bullying (Hunt & Jensen, 2007). Overall, 65% reported that they had been bullied because of their sexual orientation (this figure increased to 75% among students attending schools linked to religious-based organizations).

More studies now indicate that a number of heterosexual youth experience bullying that is homophobic (Pascoe, 2007; Poteat et al., 2011; Swearer, Turner, Givens, & Pollack, 2008). Among over 17,000 youth in Wisconsin and over 600,000 youth in California, Russell and colleagues (Russell, Sinclair, Poteat, & Koenig, 2012) found that 15.5% of youth in Wisconsin and 10.2% of youth in California reported bullying based on their actual or perceived LGB identity. Another survey among 237,544 students in California schools found that 7.5% of students had been victims of bullying on the grounds of their actual or perceived sexual orientation, while two-thirds of students who identified as LGBT reported having been victimized (O'Shaughnessy, Russell, Heck, Calhoun, & Laub, 2004). Finally, even more expansive efforts to pool representative data across the U.S. have shown sexual orientation-based victimization disparities (Russell et al., 2014).

Mental Health Disparities and Concerns Among LGBTQ Youth

As noted, LGBTQ youth face higher rates of victimization than heterosexual youth, which contributes to a range of mental, behavioral, and physical health concerns. For instance, there is strong evidence of sexual orientation-based disparities on depression, anxiety, and substance use (Almeida, Johnson, Corliss, Molnar, & Azrael, 2009; Corliss, Rosario, Wypij, Fisher, & Austin, 2008; Marshal et al., 2012; Mustanski, Garofalo, & Emerson, 2010). Meta-analyses show that these disparities are robust (Marshal et al., 2008, 2011). LGBTQ youth are at particular risk for alcohol and cigarette use (Corliss et al., 2008; Marshal et al., 2008, 2011). These factors all ultimately heighten suicidality risks; LGBTQ youth report more suicidal ideation and attempts than heterosexual youth (Marshal et al., 2011; Russell & Toomey, 2012).

Several studies have examined the prolonged effects of homophobic victimization. Prior victimization predicts subsequent suicidal ideation in LGBTQ youth (Liu & Mustanski, 2012), distress among LGBTQ and heterosexual youth (Robinson, Espelage, & Rivers, 2013), and increased anxiety among heterosexual male youth (Poteat, Scheer, DiGiovanni, & Mereish, 2014). These findings strongly suggest that the effects of homophobic victimization are not temporary or passing. Consequently, youth may need more than just immediate or temporary mental health services to address the concerns arising from homophobic victimization.

It is critical for researchers, educators, and interventionists to consider the diversity within the broader LGBTQ youth community. In one sense, this necessitates attention to specific sexual orientation or gender identities, such as lesbian, gay, bisexual, queer, or transgender youth, and the similarities and differences in experiences of youth across these specific groups. In another sense, it is important to consider the many other social identities of LGBTQ youth and how they intersect with their sexual orientation and gender identities. Certain groups of LGBTQ youth, such as youth of color, are often underrepresented in research and mental health services. Yet, these youth also face additional or unique sets of stressors that could lead to even more pronounced mental health concerns. LGBTQ youth of color may face racial discrimination in addition to sexual orientation-based discrimination (Balsam, Huang, Fieland, Simoni, & Walters, 2004; Rosario, Schrimshaw, & Hunter, 2004). Transgender youth experience frequent victimization that is associated with greater health risks (Aspenlieder, Buchanan, McDougall, & Sippola, 2009; Toomey, McGuire, & Russell, 2012) and they also face unique barriers and types of hostility within schools (e.g., not being referred to by their preferred gender pronouns or name corresponding with their affirmed gender; being prohibited from participating on the sports teams or accessing the bathrooms or locker rooms of their affirmed gender). Still other populations of LGBTQ youth remain neglected in research and practice. For instance, there is little research on LGBTQ youth with disabilities (Harley, Nowak, Gassaway, & Savage, 2002). Thus, even with the sizable literature base on the victimization of LGBTQ youth, there remain many areas in need of greater attention.

School-based Resources and Settings

School-based professionals have a responsibility to understand and take action in bolstering resilience among LGBTQ youth. Despite ongoing experiences of victimization and social stigma, LGBTQ youth indeed develop individual strengths and resilience to overcome these challenges. Disparities faced by LGBTQ youth in schools may be ameliorated by addressing the range of contributors to these disparities and by creating a welcoming and safe school environment with opportunities for LGBTQ youth to feel connected to others. In the next two sections, we review several school-based resources, policies, and approaches that could promote resilience among LGBTQ youth.

Gay-Straight Alliances

Gay-Straight Alliances (GSAs) are school-based groups that serve a critical role in fostering resilience and promoting positive development among LGBTQ youth members. Based on positive youth development models (Shinn & Yoshikawa, 2008), GSAs are intended to cultivate youths' individual strengths and to foster healthy development as youth-led and advisor-supported settings. GSAs provide safety and support, opportunities to socialize, and encourage civic engagement through advocacy and other forms of school and community engagement (Griffin, Lee, Waugh, & Beyer, 2004; Mayberry, 2006; Russell & McGuire, 2008; Russell, Muraco, Subramaniam, & Laub, 2009). In general, a growing number of studies have shown that many LGBTQ youth who participate in GSAs or who are in schools with GSAs report better health and academic outcomes (Griffin et al., 2004; Poteat et al., 2015; Walls, Kane, & Wisneski, 2010). These empirical findings indicate that GSAs can indeed serve as a school-based protective setting that promotes LGBTQ youths' mental health. Given these findings, educators, counselors, and interventionists should be aware of GSAs as an important resource.

Extracurricular Settings in General

While GSAs may play a major role in promoting the health and well-being of LGBTQ youth, it is equally important to consider the benefits of extracurricular settings in general. Structured activities encourage discipline, engagement, and skill-building, and they help youth establish social networks with peers and adults (Denault & Poulin, 2009; Fredricks & Eccles, 2006; Larson 2000; Mahoney & Stattin 2000). Youth participation in extracurricular activities has been linked to numerous positive outcomes, including higher self-esteem, lower depression, and greater psychosocial well-being (Barber, Eccles, & Stone, 2001; Libbey, 2004; Mahoney, Harris, & Eccles, 2006).

Building on these findings from the general youth programs literature, involvement in school-based extracurricular activities (e.g., sports, the arts, or other school-based clubs) could help protect LGBTQ youth against the effects of negative school experiences (Toomey et al., 2012). Extracurricular involvement could increase LGBTQ youths' sense of belonging to their school by enhancing self-worth and agency and by improving social competence. At the same time, several issues of concern must be addressed in some of these settings. For instance, although sports involvement can promote health on a number of indices, sports clubs are often hostile climates for LGBTQ youth (Gill, Morrow, Collins, Lucey, & Schultz, 2010). Therefore, school administrators and educators should continue to work to make extracurricular settings more affirming of and accessible to LGBTQ youth.

School Policies, Curriculum, and Training

A growing emphasis has been placed on several institutional and macro-level factors that are important in promoting safer and more welcoming schools and in reducing health disparities faced by LGBTQ youth. Researchers and policy experts have highlighted the importance of nondiscrimination and anti-bullying policies, inclusive curricula, ongoing educational training, and school-based resources for LGBTQ students as integral to promoting safer schools (Horn, Szalacha, & Drill, 2008; Russell, Kosciw, Horn, & Saewyc, 2010). We discuss several potential pathways through which policies and practices at this broader level may come to exert an effect on the individual experiences of LGBTQ youth at school.

Anti-Bullying and Anti-Discrimination Policies

Although there has been a proliferation of anti-bullying policies in schools, only recently have some policies included enumeration that is explicit in its protection of minority or stigmatized groups (e.g., LGBTQ youth) who historically have faced disproportionately higher rates of victimization (Russell et al., 2010). Now, there is emerging work to show that LGBTQ youth who live in districts with anti-bullying policies that enumerate the protection of sexual minorities report lower suicide risk than youth who live in districts without these enumerated policies (Hatzenbuehler & Keyes, 2013). The passage of these policies and their association with student health outcomes is encouraging; at the same time, ongoing efforts must be made to identify the specific pathways by which they lead to improved safety and health for LGBTQ youth. Identifying these pathways would provide valuable data on how these policies can be implemented most effectively. For instance, these policies may raise greater awareness of homophobic harassment, stimulate deeper discussions of these issues among educators, provide guidelines and useful strategies for how adults at school can address homophobic harassment, and prompt adults to intervene more consistently when it occurs. Nevertheless, these policies can be met with hostility (Horn et al., 2008; Russell et al., 2010). Hostility and other barriers to these policies (e.g., a lack of personal endorsement of these policies by school administrators) could reduce the fidelity with which these policies are implemented. In essence, these policies may have less of an impact on LGBTQ students' experiences when they are inconsistently enforced or are poorly applied in a given school. All of these factors, whether they may serve to facilitate or impede the application of these policies, should be considered in greater detail.

Inclusive Curricula

In addition to policies aimed at the reduction and prevention of homophobic harassment, scholars have pointed to the role of inclusive curricula (e.g., using materials that represent LGBTQ issues and individuals) in promoting welcoming schools. This approach could play as equally important a role as anti-bullying and anti-discrimination policies. Students who attend schools with inclusive curricula report greater perceptions of school safety (Russell, Kostroski, McGuire, Laub, & Manke, 2006). Similar to the attention given to anti-bullying policies, researchers must consider the pathways by which inclusive curricula may decrease homophobic harassment and increase well-being among LGBTQ youth. For instance, representation of LGBTQ individuals and issues in the standard course material may address a major obstacle that many LGBTQ youth face in school around invisibility (Chesir-Teran, 2003). The inclusion of LGBTQ issues within the standard curriculum also may send a clear signal to students that the school actively affirms and respects LGBTQ diversity. Further, it may reduce homophobic harassment and increase respect for LGBTQ students by providing important opportunities for learning and for dialogue among students about these issues and behaviors. As part of addressing these issues, research is needed to identify best practices for delivering this curriculum to maximize its effectiveness.

Adult Trainings and Continuing Education

Ongoing educator and counselor trainings are integral to reducing homophobic harassment in schools and addressing the needs of LGBTQ youth. Educators, counselors, and other adults at school are in an influential position to promote change by establishing respectful classroom norms, modeling appropriate behavior, teaching inclusive curricula, creating space for and facilitating dialogue among students, and intervening when harassment occurs. To do each of these tasks effectively, adults at school must have adequate training and opportunities to develop and practice these skills, be provided tools and materials, and feel supported in their efforts. Various training models have been proposed and materials have been generated to address sexual orientation and gender identity issues (GLSEN, n.d.; GSA Network, n.d.; Ollis, 2013; Rivers, Duncan, & Besag, 2007). Many of these trainings include coverage of basic terminology, reviewing relevant policies and procedures, building self-awareness and knowledge related to sexual orientation and gender identity and expression, and learning and practicing new skills (e.g., ways to intervene when harassment occurs, delivering curriculum, or responding to common student questions). As the number of trainings and available materials continue to grow, there is an increased need to test their immediate and long-term effectiveness. To date, it is unclear what components of these trainings, or the methods by which they are delivered, produce meaningful change and improvement in students' experiences.

Conclusions

Collaborative efforts among researchers, practitioners, and policy makers have led to advances in addressing the needs of LGBTQ youth in schools and countering the homophobic harassment that they experience in this context. Still, much remains to be done in this area in order to sustain these gains while also addressing other barriers, stressors, and needs faced by these youth. These ongoing efforts must recognize the diversity within the LGBTQ youth community and the unique needs among various groups of LGBTQ youth. This approach will ensure that resources and interventions are tailored to meet these varied needs and that they will be responsive to LGBTQ youths' other social identities that shape their experiences. Ongoing efforts must also seek to change the broader school climate and structure to be one that is affirming and welcoming of LGBTQ youth. Even more broadly, wraparound services that attend to the experiences and needs of LGBTQ youth beyond the immediate school context and across multiple other contexts are needed. This advance would better acknowledge and attend to the overlap and influence of LGBTQ youths' experiences across contexts (e.g., meeting the mental health and academic needs of an LGBTQ youth who has faced family rejection). Each of these steps will be important in continuing to advance toward the goal of ensuring the safety of LGBTQ youth, their well-being and healthy development, and access to opportunities for learning and academic achievement in schools.

Take-Home Points

- Many LGBTQ youth continue to experience chronic homophobic victimization in schools.
- The effects of homophobic victimization are prolonged; youth may need more than just immediate or temporary mental health services to address concerns related to these experiences.
- Researchers and interventionists must consider the diversity within the broader LGBTQ youth community in order to tailor their prevention and intervention efforts.
- GSAs and potentially other school-based extracurricular settings may be important resources for promoting resilience among LGBTQ youth.
- Enumerated anti-bullying policies and inclusive curricula may foster a more welcoming climate and promote safety and health among LGBTQ youth under optimal circumstances.

Resources

There are a growing number of student and adult resources for addressing issues of diversity, countering homophobic behavior, and promoting welcoming spaces for LGBTQ youth in schools. Although formal program evaluations are needed, several resources are freely available through organizations such as GLSEN (www.glsen.org) and GSA Network (www.gsanetwork.org). Other LGBTQ-supportive organizations include The Trevor Project (www.thetrevorproject.org), the Safe

Schools Coalition (www.safeschoolscoalition.org), the Family Acceptance Project (www.familyproject.sfsu.edu), and PFLAG (www.pflag.org).

References

Almeida, J., Johnson, R.M., Corliss, H.L., Molnar, B.E., & Azrael, D. (2009). Emotional distress among LGBT youth: The influence of perceived discrimination based on sexual orientation. *Journal of Youth and Adolescence, 38*, 1001–1014.

Aspenlieder, L., Buchanan, C.M., McDougall, P., & Sippola, L.K. (2009). Gender non-conformity and peer victimization in pre- and early adolescence. *European Journal of Developmental Science, 3*, 3–16.

Balsam, K.F., Huang, B., Fieland, K.C., Simoni, J.M., & Walters, K.L. (2004). Culture, trauma, and wellness: A comparison of heterosexual and lesbian, gay, bisexual, and two-spirit Native Americans. *Cultural Diversity and Ethnic Minority Psychology, 10*, 287–301.

Barber, B.L., Eccles, J.S., & Stone, M.R. (2001). Whatever happened to the "Jock," the "Brain," and the "Princess"?: Young adult pathways linked to adolescent activity involvement and social identity. *Journal of Adolescent Research, 16*, 429–455.

Berrill, K.T. (1992). Anti-gay violence and victimization in the United States: An overview. In G.M. Herek, & K.T. Berrill (Eds.), *Hate crimes: Confronting violence against lesbians and gay men* (pp. 19–45). Newbury Park: Sage.

Birkett, M., Russell, S.T., & Corliss, H.L. (2014). Sexual orientation disparities in school: The mediational role of indicators of victimization in achievement and truancy because of feeling unsafe. *American Journal of Public Health, 104*, 1124–1128.

Bronfenbrenner, U., & Morris, P.A. (2006). The bioecological model of human development. In R.M. Lerner (Ed.), *Handbook of child psychology, Vol. 1: theoretical models of human development* (6th ed., pp. 793–828). Hoboken, NJ: Wiley.

Chesir-Teran, D. (2003). Conceptualizing and addressing heterosexism in high schools: A setting-level approach. *American Journal of Community Psychology, 31*, 269–279.

Coker, T.R., Austin, S.B., & Schuster, M.A. (2010). The health and health care of lesbian, gay, and bisexual adolescents. *Annual Review of Public Health, 31*, 457–477.

Corliss, H.L., Rosario, M., Wypij, D., Fisher, L.B., & Austin, S.B. (2008). Sexual orientation disparities in longitudinal alcohol use patterns among adolescents: Findings from the Growing Up Today Study. *Archives of Pediatric and Adolescent Medice, 162*, 1071–1078.

Denault, A., & Poulin, F., (2009). Intensity and breadth of participation in organized activities during the adolescent years: Multiple associations with youth outcomes. *Journal of Youth and Adolescence, 38*, 1199–1213.

Ellis, V., & High, S. (2004). Something more to tell you: Gay, lesbian or bisexual young people's experiences of secondary schooling. *British Educational Research Journal, 30*, 213–225.

Fredricks, J.A., & Eccles, J.S. (2006). Is extracurricular participation associated with beneficial outcomes? Concurrent and longitudinal relations. *Developmental Psychology, 42*, 698–713.

Gay, Lesbian, and Straight Education Network (GLSEN). (n.d.). Educator resources. Retrieved from http://www.glsen.org/educate/resources

Gill, D.L., Morrow, R.G., Collins, K.E., Lucey, A.B., & Schultz, A.M. (2010). Perceived climate in physical activity settings. *Journal of Homosexuality, 57*, 895–913.

Griffin, P., Lee, C., Waugh, J., & Beyer, C. (2004). Describing roles that gay-straight alliances play in schools: From individual support to school change. *Journal of Gay & Lesbian Issues in Education, 1*, 7–22.

Gross, L., Aurand. S., & Adessa, R. (1988). *Violence and discrimination against lesbian and gay people in Philadelphia and the Commonwealth of Pennsylvania*. Philadelphia: Philadelphia Lesbian and Gay Task Force.

Grossman, A.H., & D'Augelli, A.R. (2006). Transgender youth: Invisible and vulnerable. *Journal of Homosexuality, 51*, 111–128.

GSA Network. (n.d.). Resources. Retrieved from http://www.gsanetwork.org/resources

Harley, D.A., Nowak, T.M., Gassaway, L.J., & Savage, T.A. (2002). Lesbian, gay, bisexual, and transgender college students with disabilities: A look at multiple cultural minorities. *Psychology in Schools, 39*, 525–538.

Hatzenbuehler, M.L., & Keyes, K.M. (2013). Inclusive anti-bullying policies and reduced risk of suicide attempts in lesbian and gay youth. *Journal of Adolescent Health, 53*, S21–S26.

Horn, S.S., Szalacha, L.A., & Drill, K. (2008). Schooling, sexuality, and rights: An investigation of heterosexual students' social cognition regarding sexual orientation and the rights of gay and lesbian peers in school. *Journal of Social Issues, 64*, 791–813.

Hunt, R., & Jensen, J. (2007). *The school report: The experiences of gay young people in Britain's schools*. London: Stonewall

Kosciw, J.G., Greytak, E.A., Bartkiewicz, M.J., Boesen, M.J., & Palmer, N.A. (2012). *The 2011 National School Climate Survey: The experiences of lesbian, gay, bisexual and transgender youth in our nation's schools*. New York: GLSEN.

Larson, R.W. (2000). Toward a psychology of positive youth development. *American Psychologist, 55*, 170–183.

Libbey, H.P. (2004). Measuring student relationships to school: Attachment, bonding, connectedness, and engagement. *Journal of School Health, 74*, 274–283.

Liu, R.T., & Mustanski, B. (2012). Suicidal ideation and self-harm in lesbian, gay, bisexual, and transgender youth. *American Journal of Preventive Medicine, 42*, 221–228.

Mahoney, J.L., Harris, A.L., & Eccles, J.S. (2006). Organized activity participation, positive youth development, and the overscheduling hypothesis. *Society for Research in Child Development: Social Policy Report, 20*, 1–30.

Mahoney, J.L., & Stattin, H. (2000). Leisure activities and adolescent antisocial behavior: The role of structure and social context. *Journal of Adolescence, 23*, 113–127.

Marshal, M.P., Dietz, L.J., Friedman, M.S., Stall, R., Smith, H.A., McGinley, J., . . . & Brent, D.A. (2011). Suicidality and depression disparities between sexual minority and heterosexual youth: A meta-analytic review. *Journal of Adolescent Health, 49*, 115–123.

Marshal, M.P., Friedman, M.S., Stall, R., King, K.M., Miles, J., Gold, M.A., . . . Morse, J.Q. (2008). Sexual orientation and adolescent substance use: A meta-analysis and methodological review. *Addiction, 103*, 546–556.

Marshal, M.P., King, K.M., Stepp, S.D., Hipwell, A., Smith, H., Chung, T., . . . Markovic, N. (2012). Trajectories of alcohol and cigarette use among sexual minority and heterosexual girls. *Journal of Adolescent Health, 50*, 97–99.

Mayberry, M. (2006). The story of a Salt Lake City gay-straight alliance: Identity work and LGBT youth. *Journal of Gay & Lesbian Issues in Education, 4*, 13–31.

Meyer, I. (2003). Prejudice, social stress, and mental health in lesbian, gay, and bisexual populations: Conceptual issues and research evidence. *Psychological Bulletin, 129*, 674–697.

Mustanski, B.S., Garofalo, R., & Emerson, E.M. (2010). Mental health disorders, psychological distress, and suicidality in a diverse sample of lesbian, gay, bisexual, and transgender youths. *American Journal of Public Health, 100*, 2426–2432.

Ollis, D. (2013). Planning and delivering intervention to promote gender and sexuality. In I. Rivers, & N. Duncan (Eds.), *Bullying: Experiences and discourses of sexuality and gender* (pp. 145–161). London: Routledge.

O'Shaughnessy, M., Russell, S.T., Heck, K., Calhoun, C., & Laub, C. ((2004). *Safe place to learn: Consequences of harassment based on actual or perceived sexual orientation and gender non-conformity and step for making schools safer.* San Francisco: California Safe Schools Coalition & 4-H Centre for Youth Development.

Pascoe, C.J. (2007). *Dude, you're a fag: Masculinity and sexuality in high school.* Los Angeles, CA: University of California Press.

Pilkington, N.W., & D'Augelli, A.R. (1995). Victimization of lesbian, gay, and bisexual youth in community settings. *Journal of Community Psychology, 23,* 33–56.

Poteat, V.P., Mereish, E.H., DiGiovanni, C.D., & Koenig, B.W. (2011). The effects of general and homophobic victimization on adolescents' psychosocial and educational concerns: The importance of intersecting identities and parent support. *Journal of Counseling Psychology, 58,* 597–609.

Poteat, V.P., Scheer, J.R., DiGiovanni, C.D., & Mereish, E.H. (2014). Short-term prospective effects of homophobic victimization on the mental health of heterosexual adolescents. *Journal of Youth and Adolescence, 43,* 1240–1251.

Poteat, V.P., Yoshikawa, H., Calzo, J.P., Gray, M.L., DiGiovanni, C.D., Lipkin, A., . . . Shaw, M.P. (2015). Contextualizing gay-straight alliances: Student, advisor, and structural factors related to positive youth development among members. *Child Development, 86,* 176–193.

Rivers, I. (2001). The bullying of sexual minorities at school: Its nature and long-term correlates. *Educational and Child Psychology, 18,* 32–46.

Rivers, I., Duncan, N., & Besag, V.E. (2007). *Bullying: A handbook for educators and parents.* Westport: Greenwood/Praeger.

Robinson, J.P., Espelage, D.L., & Rivers, I. (2013). Developmental trends in peer victimization and emotional distress in LGB and heterosexual youth. *Pediatrics, 131,* 423–430.

Rosario, M., Schrimshaw, E.W., & Hunter, J. (2004). Ethnic/racial differences in the coming-out process of lesbian, gay, and bisexual youths: A comparison of sexual identity development over time. *Cultural Diversity and Ethnic Minority Psychology, 10,* 215–228.

Russell, S.T., Everett, B.G., Rosario, M., & Birkett, M. (2014). Indicators of victimization and sexual orientation among adolescents: Analyses from youth risk behavior surveys. *American Journal of Public Health, 104,* 255–261. doi: 10.2105/AJPH.2013.301493

Russell, S.T., Kosciw, J., Horn, S., & Saewyc, E. (2010). Safe schools policy for LGBTQ students. *Society for Research in Child Development Social Policy Report, 24,* 3–17.

Russell, S.T., Kostroski, O., McGuire, J.K., Laub, C., & Manke, E. (2006). *LGBT issues in the curriculum promotes school safety.* California Safe Schools Coalition Research Brief No. 4. San Francisco, CA: California Safe Schools Coalition.

Russell, S.T., & McGuire, J.K. (2008). The school climate for lesbian, gay, bisexual, and transgender (LGBT) students. In M. Shinn & H. Yoshikawa (Eds.), *Toward positive youth development: Transforming schools and community programs* (pp. 133–149). New York: Oxford University Press.

Russell, S.T., Muraco, A., Subramaniam, A., & Laub, C. (2009). Youth empowerment and high school gay-straight alliances. *Journal of Youth and Adolescence, 38,* 891–903.

Russell, S.T., Sinclair, K.O., Poteat, V.P., & Koenig, B.W. (2012). Adolescent health and harassment based on discriminatory bias. *American Journal of Public Health, 102,* 493–495.

Russell, S.T., & Toomey, R.B. (2012). Men's sexual orientation and suicide: Evidence for U.S. adolescent-specific risk. *Social Science and Medicine, 74,* 523–529.

Shinn, M., & Yoshikawa, H. (2008). *Toward positive youth development: Transforming schools and community programs.* New York: Oxford University Press.

Swearer, S.M., Turner, R.K., Givens, J.E., & Pollack, W.S. (2008). "You're so gay!" Do different forms of bullying matter for adolescent males? *School Psychology Review*, *37*, 160–173.

Toomey, R.B., McGuire, J.K., & Russell, S.T. (2012). Heteronormativity, school climates, and perceived safety for gender nonconforming peers. *Journal of Adolescence*, *35*, 187–196.

Walls, N.E., Kane, S., B., & Wisneski, H. (2010). Gay–straight alliances and school experiences of sexual minority youth. *Youth & Society*, *41*, 307–332.

11

FAMILY ADJUSTMENT ISSUES

Cheryl Buehler and Kamilah B. Legette

Families and schools are important microsystems for the developing child and the family-school interface is an influential mesosystem in the child's life (Rogers, Theule, Ryan, Adams, & Keating, 2009). In this chapter, we focus on three aspects of family life that may influence how children and youth navigate their school experiences: cumulative family risk, family demography, and parental functioning.

Cumulative Family Risk

A cumulative risk perspective suggests that it is the *accumulation* of environmental risk factors that jeopardizes children's/youth's well-being rather than the experience of a particular stressor (Buehler & Gerard, 2013). This chapter focuses on cumulative *family* risk and various markers of children's educational and school adjustment.

During the first nine years of life, language difficulties and children's school behavior problems demonstrate moderately strong associations with the *accumulation* of family risk factors, including poverty, low parental educational status, high maternal depressive symptoms, poor mother-child interactions, and low home environment quality (Deater-Deckard, Dodge, Bates, & Pettit, 1998; Stanton-Chapman, Chapman, Kaiser, & Hancock, 2004). In middle school, youths' academic (Buehler & Gerard, 2013; Gutman, Sameroff, & Eccles, 2002), behavioral (Loukas, Prelow, Suizzo, & Allua, 2008), and emotional difficulties (Parra, DuBois, & Sher, 2006) are also associated with the *accumulation* of family risk, with risk factors including low maternal educational status, single parenthood, low family income, mothers' psychological distress, parents' life dissatisfaction, parent-adolescent relationship problems, marital hostility, and triangulating the child in marital disputes. Samples from these studies were diverse in terms of race, ethnicity, marital status, and socioeconomic status, with robust school-related effects found even in a sample of two-parent, European American families, which is a group of families that often is viewed as a relatively monolithic and insulated configuration in terms of family risk. Further, in high school the *accumulation* of various family risk factors—including single-parent status, low income, parental unemployment, limited English proficiency, low family warmth and connection, and parent-youth conflict—have been linked to not completing high school, behavior problems, and elevated depressive symptoms (Matjasko, Grunden, & Ernst, 2007; Van Dorn, Bowen, & Blau, 2006). Finally, three longitudinal studies that examined cumulative family risk from when children were young also have shown difficulties when youth are in high school (Appleyard, Egeland, van Dulmen, & Sroufe, 2005; Gutman, Sameroff, & Cole, 2003; Smokowski, Mann, Reynolds, & Fraser, 2004), providing strong evidence that the *accumulation* of family risk factors creates vulnerabilities for children/youth as they progress from elementary school through high school.

Family Demography

Family demographic factors may be important for children's school experiences because they affect familial resources, expectations, aspirations, and experiences, as well as play an integral role in nesting children in various ecological niches that shape opportunities and risks.

Socioeconomic Status

There is a robust association between family SES and students' school-related outcomes (Chiu & Chow, 2015). A meta-analysis on literature through the 1970s documented that the average correlation across studies between particular SES components and student academic achievement was .32 for income, .20 for parents' occupational status, and .19 for parental education (White, 1982). Focusing on parental educational attainment only, mothers' schooling or additional schooling after the child is born facilitates children's school readiness and success in school (Kingston, Huang, Calzada, Dawson-McClure, & Brotman, 2013; Magnuson, 2007). Although these associations tend to be fairly weak to moderate in strength, effects may be stronger and more influential when intersected with family structure, race, or ethnicity.

Hoff (2013) has argued that family SES differences impact early language development in important ways (i.e., vocabulary size, grammatical development, narrative skills) that shape young children's early school success and ultimately affect academic trajectories through high school. A recent meta-analysis has shown that these early language and reading skills are strong predictors of later academic achievement for students with both high and low family SES (Duncan et al., 2007). Primary-school teachers' perceptions of students' academic capacities help explain how family adversity such as low SES places children at greater risk for difficulties in school (Gut, Reimann, & Grob, 2013), documenting the interplay between home and school factors.

The inverse association between family SES and children's academic achievement extends to secondary school (Buehler & Gerard, 2013) and beyond. In a large sample of middle-school students, free/reduced school lunch status (FRSL) was not associated with school engagement, but was associated with lower grades and lower levels of trouble avoidance in school (Bowen, Rose, Powers, & Glennie, 2008). Further, data from the National Educational Longitudinal Study (NELS) documented a positive association between family SES and high school test scores, controlling for race, 10th grade GPA, cultural capital, social capital, student academic engagement, teacher perceptions of student performance, and school quality (Oates, 2009). Finally, family SES may have long-term effects on young adults' educational attainment; a recent study found that high school guidance counselors recommended community college to students from lower SES backgrounds but 4-year higher education to students from higher SES backgrounds (Linnehan, Weer, & Stonely, 2011).

Race and Ethnicity

We only briefly review some of the voluminous literature on student race/ethnicity and school-related outcomes, particularly as issues relate to family factors. As summarized by Bali and Alvarez (2003), the Black-White achievement gap has been decreasing over several decades but test scores continue to favor White students by almost a standard deviation. A gap in test scores also exists between Hispanic and White students, "with a gap larger than the black-white test gap in reading, but smaller in math" (Bali & Alvarez, 2003, p. 486).

Students' academic achievement, feelings about school, emotional distress, and avoidance of trouble at school are firmly nested in family, neighborhood, and school contexts in complex and nuanced ways. Grogan-Kaylor and Woolley (2010) examined the social ecology of race and ethnic school achievement gaps, analyzing data from a large, representative sample of youth in middle and high school. They found that student-reported grades were lower for African American, Latino, Native American, and students of "other races" than for White students. These racial and ethnic differences disappeared for African American and Latino students when family sociodemographic factors were considered. They also studied students' avoidance of problem behaviors in school and found that African American students reported greater trouble avoidance than did White students. Finally, they considered school coherence, defined as youth liking school, being able to make sense out of school, and being able to identify success strategies. African American, multiracial, and "other" students reported higher levels of school coherence than did White students. This latter finding is consistent with recent research that has shown that African American students tend to be more engaged academically than are White students (Bowen et al., 2008; Oates, 2009). Using the NELS data when students were in 10th and 12th grades, Oates concluded that the racial achievement gap is best explained by what happens to students when they are at school rather than by explanations that center around what students bring to school (like their family experiences). More specifically, she found that the Black-White achievement gap is best explained by differences in school quality and by biased treatment by teachers. Condron and colleagues also examined school factors and found that racial segregation (i.e., dissimilarity scores) and Black student isolation contribute to the Black-White achievement gap, whereas increased exposure of Black students to White students diminished the gap (Condron, Tope, Steidl, & Freeman, 2012).

Immigration Status

Child and parental immigration status also is associated with students' academic achievement. Some research has documented advantages (labeled the immigration educational paradox), whereas other research has documented disadvantages (labeled the immigration achievement gap). Simms (2012) analyzed achievement test scores from kindergarten through 8th grade using data on 6,861 students from the ECLS-K. She found that immigrant students had lower math scores when they began kindergarten than did nonimmigrant students. Children born in other countries who immigrated before age 6 caught up to nonimmigrant children in math achievement by 8th grade, but children born in the U.S. to an immigrant mother did not. She found that nationality better explained achievement gaps than did race.

Simms (2012) and Hoff (2013) note that immigrant children's school success is influenced by their English language proficiency. Hoff reviewed literature that suggests that school readiness is lower for low-income bilingual children than for middle-class monolingual children. She notes that children's early experiences with books in their first language facilitates reading comprehension skills in their second language, highlighting again, in this different context, the importance of parenting practices that involve books, reading together, and verbal conversations. Hoff contended that immigrant children need extra support for the development of needed English skills, "while also valuing and making use of children's home language skills" (p. 11).

Family Structure

There has been a longstanding interest in the interconnections between family structure and children's school-related outcomes. As with family SES, race and ethnicity, and immigration status, issues surrounding family structure and children's school experiences are complex in that they invoke societal stratifications and constraints, as well as parental and coparental stresses and capacities. Amato

(2001) conducted a meta-analysis of research published during the 1990s and found a significant correlation between parental *divorce* and children's academic achievement (favoring married families). In a more recent study, Zeiders and colleagues compared two-parent and single-parent Mexican American families (Zeiders, Roosa, & Tein, 2011). Early adolescents in single-parent families had greater levels of school misconduct, general conduct problems, and depressive symptoms, and these differences with married families were explained by greater family stress and parent-child hostile conflict.

In a meta-analysis of studies published through the mid 2000s (Jeynes, 2006) that focused on parental *remarriage*, results indicated that the average association with overall school behavior and academic achievement favored children in first-marriage families. Children living in remarried families had lower scores on psychological well-being than did children in first-marriage families, and lower scores than did children living in single-parent families, but this difference was not statistically significant.

One of the structural issues receiving increased attention has addressed complexities surrounding parental *cohabitation*. Brown (2004) analyzed data from the 1999 National Survey of America's Families (N = 35,938) found that children aged 6 to 11 living in cohabitating families (both birth and step) had lower school engagement scores than did children living in two biological married families. These differences remained when including various measures of economic and parental resources.

Researchers have begun to examine how *changes* in family structure are associated with various child outcomes. Ram and Hou (2003) analyzed three waves of data from the National Longitudinal Surveys of Children and Youth and found that changing from a two-parent, married family to a single-parent or remarried family was associated with lower child well-being. They also found that family economic resources were most useful for explaining difference in children's cognitive difficulties, whereas ineffective parenting and parental depressive symptoms were most useful for explaining children's emotional and behavioral difficulties. Fomby and Cherlin (2007) used data from two large national datasets to examine how multiple changes in family structure are associated with children's cognitive and behavioral difficulties (children aged 5–14). They found no robust effects of multiple structural transitions for African American children's cognitive or behavioral outcomes but an inverse association for European American children's outcomes. Future research on children's school-related outcomes needs to continue this ecological contextualization by considering these various intersections among family SES, race, ethnicity, children's birth status, and family structure.

Employment (Including Military Families)

Research exploring the relationship between parental employment, particularly maternal employment, and child outcomes has found inconsistent and nonsignificant results. Goldberg, Prause, Lucas-Thompson, and Himsel (2008) examined the association between maternal employment and children's academic achievement by conducting a meta-analysis of 68 studies. They found that there was no significant overall association between employment and child academic achievement, but that the association differed when considering the moderating effects of family SES, race/ethnicity, and family structure. Specifically, there were more academic benefits associated with maternal employment for working/lower middle class children compared to middle/upper middle class children, for racially/ethnically diverse samples than for White samples, and for samples with only one parent than for samples with only two-parents.

Research examining children in military families has focused on parental deployment and geographic mobility. Parental deployment has been associated with lower test scores, increased internalizing and externalizing symptoms, and child maltreatment (Chartrand, Frank, White, & Shope, 2008; Engel, Gallagher, & Lyle, 2010; Gibbs, Martin, Kupper, & Johnson, 2007). Geographic mobility also is a concern because a typical military family moves every two to three years (Park, 2011). Youth report that constantly changing schools and leaving friends are highly stressful experiences (Leitzel, Charlton, & Jeffreys, 1997). These experiences have been associated with more school-related difficulties and emotional and behavior problems, such as feelings of loneliness, isolation, and depression (Ashby, 2003).

Parental Functioning

We use the ecologically based Family-School Relationships Model to frame our review of the voluminous literature on parenting (Rogers et al., 2009). This set of nested levels of influence suggests that child behaviors or accomplishments are shaped by children's traits and competencies, school-focused parent-child interactions, general parent-child interactions, general family relations (including marital/coparental functioning), personal characteristics of parents (including psychological well-being), and exogenous social/cultural variables (e.g., neighborhood features, teachers, peers). Much, but not all of this research, has focused on mothers' parenting.

Young Children's Learning and School Readiness

School readiness includes motivation to learn, task persistence, receptive vocabulary skills, and social-emotional competencies. Fantuzzo, McWayne, Perry, and Childs (2004) found that home-based involvement (i.e., creating and using home learning environments) was an important correlate with young children's learning motivation, task persistence, and vocabulary skills. Home- and school-based involvement worked together to minimize conduct problems at school. Findings with a similar sample of Head Start families supported the importance of both home- and school-based parenting practices for kindergartener's academic and social competencies (McWayne, Hampton, Fantuzzo, Cohen, & Sekino, 2004). In line with the Family-School Relationships model, reading-oriented parenting practices during toddlerhood have been associated with school readiness at age 5, and this association was partly due to increased expressive language skills (Forget-Dubois et al., 2009).

Several studies have examined the role of parenting in children's school readiness in diverse racial and ethnic samples of families. Using data from the ECLS-K, Raver, Gershoff, and Aber (2007) found that an aggregate of home- and school-based parenting practices (they termed parental investment) was associated with higher child cognitive skills at age 6. This association was positive and similar in strength for Black, Hispanic, and White families. They also found a positive association between positive parenting behavior (assessed via warmth, cognitive stimulation, lower use of physical punishment, use of facilitating rules and routines) and child social-emotional competence. This association was stronger for White families than for families of color, but significant in each group.

Elementary School

In their test of the Family-School Relationships model, Rogers et al. (2009) examined mothers' and fathers' parenting practices in relation to 5th and 6th graders' academic achievement. Mothers' active management of the learning environment, their encouragement and support for learning, and their participation with homework were each uniquely associated with children's academic achievement via children's higher levels of perceived academic competence. After controlling for these factors, the unique, direct effect of participation with homework with academic achievement was negative. Help with homework may have both supportive and intrusive/demanding components. Fathers' active management of the learning environment also was associated positively with children's achievement through child perceived academic competence. Academic pressure and participation had negative associations with achievement through lower levels of perceived child academic competence. Barnard's (2004) finding that teacher ratings of parents' school involvement were associated with better school success also suggests that finding ways to remove barriers for low-income parents' school involvement may have long-term salutary effects.

Middle School

In their meta-analysis of 50 studies, Hill and Tyson (2009) documented an average weighted effect size of .18 ($p < .05$) between various aspects of parental involvement and youths' academic achievement. They examined three types of parental involvement: home-based, school-based, and academic socialization. During middle school, parental involvement via academic socializations (e.g., discussing expectations, utility, and success strategies) had the strongest association with achievement (.39). Helping with homework (part of home-based involvement) was associated with lower academic achievement, whereas other home-based activities were associated with higher achievement (.12). This study of the existing literature suggests that academic socialization is an important parenting practice that support programs need to address and distinguish from home- and school-based parental involvement.

As with the literature review on young children's school readiness, supportive/enriching parenting and language skills also shape the interconnections between social risk (e.g., poverty, parental depressive symptoms, low school quality) and youths' success during the transition into middle school. Burchinal, Roberts, Zeisel, and Rowley (2008) followed African American children as they progressed from 4th through 6th grades. They found that social risk (4th grade) was associated with lower math scores and higher externalizing behavior problems (6th grade). In support of the Family-School Relationships model, language skills mediated the association between risk and math achievement. Instead of mediation, though, language skills buffered some of the deleterious effects of risk on reading achievement. Anticipation of racial discrimination exacerbated the negative effects of social risk on achievement and school-related behavior problems. Emotionally and cognitively supportive parenting were associated with better outcomes during the transition into middle school, but did not mediate or moderate the effects of social risk.

The importance of parental investments in the home learning environment for children's success during secondary school is highlighted by a recent analysis of data from the National Education Longitudinal Survey. Altschul (2011) examined various forms of parental involvement in Mexican American children's education during 8th and 10th grade. She found that involvement mattered for youths' 8th grade test scores, which then affected 10th grade test scores. Parental practices that created an enriching and supportive learning environment were associated with higher test scores, whereas help with homework was associated with lower test scores.

In addition to specific parenting practices focused on educational outcomes, general parenting behavior also is associated with children's academic success during middle school. Buehler and Gerard (2013) constructed a parenting risk index of low maternal warmth, higher maternal harshness, low paternal warmth, and higher paternal harshness. They found that parenting risk was associated with lower grades, controlling for risk in three additional family domains (marital, sociodemographic, parental psychological).

High School

One of the classic cross-sectional studies of parenting and youth's academic and social success during high school compared authoritative and nonauthoritative parenting (i.e., parenting styles) across 16 ecological niches that intersected race/ethnicity, SES, and family marital structure (Steinberg, Mounts, Lamborn, & Dornbusch, 1991). Across the majority of niches, youth with authoritative parents had higher GPAs, greater self-reliance, lower psychological distress, and less delinquency than did youth with nonauthoritative parents. However, there were niches in which parenting styles were not associated with these youth outcomes, including 50% of the niches for African American and Asian families. Parenting styles did not differ in about 38% of the niches in Hispanic families and 13% of the niches in European American families. Additional analyses of these data found that the specific parenting practices of parental school involvement and encouragement in educational engagement were more effective in promoting youths' school-related success in the general context of authoritative parenting than non-authoritative parenting (Steinberg, Lamborn, Dornbusch, & Darling, 1992).

Parent-adolescent conflict also has been a focus of parenting research and school-related outcomes during high school. Dotterer, Hoffman, Crouter, and McHale (2008) studied predominantly White, middle and working class, two-parent families across two years. They found that the frequency of parent-adolescent conflict was associated with declines in achievement over two years of high school. They also found reciprocal effects, such that lower math grades predicted increased parent-adolescent conflict two years later. This suggests that parents continue to have expectations for academic achievement during high school and that some may struggle during this period to support their children's agency and success.

There has been continued interest in the intersections among race, parenting, and youths' school-related outcomes. Somers and colleagues (2011) examined parental involvement (assessed as time spent together) in a relatively large sample of urban African American youth aged 14. Time spent together between fathers and their adolescent children mediated the association between maternal substance problems and youth grades. This finding supported the Family School Relationships model, which suggests that parenting is a more proximal family factor than parent's individual adjustment, and highlighted the potential importance of fathering. Bean, Bush, McKenry, and Wilson (2003) examined the association between three general parenting behaviors and youth functioning in African American and European American high schoolers: parental support, behavioral control, and psychological control. They found support for the importance of each of these parenting behaviors with differences occurring by race and gender of parent.

Racial/Ethnic Socialization

There is a growing literature on the role of parents' racial/ethnic socialization and children's school-related outcomes. We endorse Barbarin and Jean-Baptiste's (2013) elaboration of the definition of parenting practices as steps parents and families take to promote children's effective functioning *within their sociocultural milieus*. When children are young, there is evidence that both parents' home-based involvement in learning and parenting practices that instill racial/ethnic pride have been associated with better behavior and higher vocabulary scores, whereas the promotion of mistrust or preparation for bias have been related to less advantageous outcomes (Caughy et al., 2002).

The importance of these nuanced distinctions in various parenting practices also may exist during school. Hughes and colleagues (2009) found that cultural socialization was associated with better student academic and behavioral outcomes during primary school, and that this association was partly due to increased ethnic affirmation and self-esteem (Hughes, Witherspoon, Rivas-Drake, & West-Bey, 2009). They also found that messages focused on preparation for bias were associated with more negative academic outcomes. During middle school, Smalls (2009) found that the parenting practice of socializing youth about potential racial barriers in school and society was associated with greater youth school engagement and task persistence *when* mothers' had a more democratic-involved parenting style. During high school, Wang and Huguley (2012) found that parental cultural socialization (assessed as racial knowledge and pride) buffered the negative effects of teacher discrimination on youths' GPA and their education aspirations. Buffering effects also were evident for the association between discrimination from peers and GPA. The parenting practice of preparation for racial bias only had salutary effects on educational aspirations when it was accompanied by higher parental cultural socialization. These studies document the complexities at the intersection of academic and racial socialization parenting practices.

Take-Home Points

- Cumulative family risk influences children who live in diverse family structures and sociocultural niches that encumber various advantages and disadvantages in opportunity structures.
- Family SES intersects with family structure, race, ethnicity, and immigration status, but SES variability influences children's school-related outcomes within these various niches.
- Family SES shapes children's school readiness, which combines with parents' continued home and school-based involvement, their academic socialization, and supports/opportunities from teachers and school counselors to affect academic and behavioral trajectories over time.
- Family SES intersects with family structure, race, ethnicity, and immigration status, but SES variability influences children's school-related outcomes within these various niches.
- Children, particularly White children, living with cohabitating coparents (birth or not) are in a particularly vulnerable niche with regards to academic achievement and conduct.
- Parenting practices that promote children's problem-solving abilities, their language skills, their task persistence, and their positive approaches to learning

seem to be particularly useful in promoting children's and youths' academic success.

- The intersectionality between academic and racial socialization is central and highlights the need for family adjustment issues and youths' academic success to be placed within a sociocultural context.

References

Altschul, I. (2011). Parental involvement and the academic achievement of Mexican American youths: What kinds of involvement in youths' education matter most? *Social Work Research, 35*, 159–170.

Amato, P.R. (2001). Children of divorce in the 1990s: An update of the Amato and Keith (1991) meta-analysis. *Journal of Family Psychology, 15*, 355–370.

Appleyard, K., Egeland, B., van Dulmen, M.H.M., & Sroufe, L.A. (2005). When more is not better: The role of cumulative risk in child behavior outcomes. *Journal of Child Psychology and Psychiatry, 46*, 235–245.

Ashby, J. (2003). Geographic mobility, family, and maternal variables as related to the psychosocial adjustment of military children. *Military Medicine, 168*.

Bali, V. A., & Alvarez, R. M. (2003). Schools and educational outcomes: What causes the "race gap" in student test scores? *Social Science Quarterly, 84*, 485–507.

Barbarin, O., & Jean-Baptiste, E. (2013). The relation of dialogic, control and racial socialization practices to early academic and social competence: Effects of gender, ethnicity, and family socioeconomic status. *American Journal of Orthopsychiatry, 83*, 207–217.

Barnard, W. M. (2004). Parent involvement in elementary school and educational attainment. *Children and Youth Services Review, 26*, 39–62.

Bean, R. A., Bush, K. R., McKenry, P. C., & Wilson, S. M. (2003). The impact of parental support, behavioral control, and psychological control on the academic achievement and self-esteem of African American and European American adolescents. *Journal of Adolescent Research, 18*, 523–541.

Bowen, G. L., Rose, R. A., Powers, J. D., & Glennie, E. J. (2008). The joint effects of neighborhoods, schools, peers, and families on changes in school success of middle school students. *Family Relations, 57*, 504–516.

Brown, S.L. (2004). Family structure and child well-being: The significance of parental cohabitation. *Journal of Marriage and Family, 66*, 351–367.

Buehler, C., & Gerard, J.M. (2013). Cumulative family risk predicts increases in adjustment difficulties across early adolescence. *Journal of Youth and Adolescence, 42*, 905–920.

Burchinal, M.R., Roberts, J.E., Zeisel, S.A., & Rowley, S.J. (2008). Social risk and protective factors for African American children's academic achievement and adjustment during the transition to middle school. *Developmental Psychology, 44*, 286–292.

Caughy, M.O., O'Campo, P.J., Randolph, S.M., & Nickerson, K. (2002). The influence of racial socialization practices on the cognitive and behavioral competence of African American preschoolers. *Child Development, 73*, 1611–1625.

Chartrand, M.M., Frank, D.A., White, L.F., & Shope, T.R. (2008). Effect of parents' wartime deployment on the behavior of young children in military families. *Archives of Pediatrics & Adolescent Medicine, 162*, 1009–1014.

Chiu, M.M., & Chow, B.W.Y. (2015). Classmates characteristics and student achievement in 33 countries: Classmates' past achievement, family socioeconomic status, educational resources, and attitudes toward reading. *Journal of Educational Psychology, 107*(1), 152–169.

Condron, D. J., Tope, D., Steidl, C. R., & Freeman, K. J. (2012). Racial segregation and the black/white achievement gap, 1992 to 2009. *The Sociological Quarterly, 54*, 130–157.

Deater-Deckard, K., Dodge, K.A., Bates, J.E., & Pettit, G.S. (1998). Multiple risk factors in the development of externalizing behavior problems: Group and individual differences. *Development and Psychopathology, 10*, 469–493. doi: 10.1017/S0954579498001709

Dotterer, A.M., Hoffman, L., Crouter, A.C., & McHale, S.M. (2008). A longitudinal examination of the bicirectional links between academic achievement and parent-adolescent conflict. *Journal of Family Issues, 29*, 762–779.

Duncan, G.J., Dowsett, C.J., Claessens, A., Magnuson, K., Huston, A.C., Klebanov, P., . . . Duckworth, K. (2007). School readiness and later achievement. *Developmental Psychology, 43*, 1428–1446.

Engel, R.C., Gallagher, L.B., & Lyle, D.S. (2010). Military deployments and children's academic achievement: Evidence from Department of Defense Education Activity Schools. *Economics of Education Review, 29*, 73–82.

Fantuzzo, J., McWayne, C., Perry, M.A., & Childs, S. (2004). Multiple dimensions of family involvement and their relations to behavioral and learning competencies for urban, low-income children. *School Psychology Review, 33*, 467–480.

Fomby, P., & Cherlin, A.J. (2007). Family instability and child well-being. *American Sociological Review, 72*, 181–204.

Forget-DuBois, N., Dionne, G., Lemelin, J.P., Perusse, D., Tremblay, R.E., & Boivin, M. (2009). Early child language mediates the relation between home environment and school readiness. *Child Development, 80*, 736–749.

Gibbs, D.A., Martin, S.L., Kupper, L.L., & Johnson, R.E. (2007). Child maltreatment in enlisted soldiers' families during combat-related deployments. *JAMA, 298*, 528–535.

Goldberg, W.A., Prause, J., Lucas-Thompson, R., & Himsel, A. (2008). Maternal employment and children's achievement in context: A meta-analysis of four decades of research. *Psychological Bulletin, 134*, 77–108.

Grogan-Kaylor, A., & Woolley, M.E. (2010). The social ecology of race and ethnicity school achievement gaps: Economic, neighborhood, school and family factors. *Journal of Human Behavior in the Social Environment, 20*, 875–896.

Gut, J., Reimann, G., & Grob, A. (2013). A contextualized view on long-term predictors of academic performance. *Journal of Educational Psychology, 105*, 436–443.

Gutman, L.M., Sameroff, A.J., & Cole, R. (2003). Academic growth curve trajectories from 1st grade to 12th grade: effects of multiple social risk factors and preschool child factors. *Developmental Psychology, 39*, 777–790.

Gutman, L. M., Sameroff, A. J., & Eccles, J. S. (2002). The academic achievement of African American students during early adolescence: An examination of multiple risk, promotive, and protective factors. *American Journal of Community Psychology, 30*, 367–399.

Hill, N.E., & Tyson, D.F. (2009). Parental involvement in middle school: A meta-analytic assessment of the strategies that promote achievement. *Developmental Psychology, 45*, 740–763.

Hoff, E. (2013). Interpreting the early language trajectories of children from low-SES and language minority homes: Implications for closing achievement gaps. *Developmental Psychology, 49*, 4–14.

Hughes, D., Witherspoon, D., Rivas-Drake, D., & West-Bey, N. (2009). Received ethnic–racial socialization messages and youths' academic and behavioral outcomes: Examining the mediating role of ethnic identity and self-esteem. *Cultural Diversity and Ethnic Minority Psychology, 15*, 112.

Jeynes, W. H. (2006). The impact of parental remarriage on children: A meta-analysis. *Marriage and Family Review, 40*(4), 75–102.

Kingston, S., Huang, K.Y., Calzada, E., Dawson-McClure, S., & Brotman, L. (2013). Parent involvement in education as a moderator of family and neighborhood socioeconomic context on school readiness among young children. *Journal of Community Psychology, 41*, 265–276.

Leiber, M., Mack, K., & Featherstone, R. (2009). Family structure, family processes, economic factors, and delinquency. *Youth Violence and Juvenile Justice, 7*, 79–99.

Leitzel, D., Charlton, N., & Jeffreys, D. (1997). A qualitative analysis of the comments of military adolescents completing a worldwide survey: MFI Tech. Rep. 97–4. Scranton, PA: Military Family Institute.

Linnehan, F., Weer, C. H., & Stonely, P. (2011). High school guidance counselor recommendations: The role of student race, socioeconomic status, and academic performance. *Journal of Applied Social Psychology, 41*, 536–558.

Loukas, A., Prelow, H. M., Suizzo, M. A., & Allua, S. (2008). Mothering and peer associations mediate cumulative risk effects for Latino youth. *Journal of Marriage and Family, 70*, 76–85.

Magnuson, K. (2007). Maternal education and children's academic achievement during middle childhood. *Developmental Psychology, 43*, 1497–1512.

Matjasko, J. L., Grunden, L. N., & Ernst, J. L. (2007). Structural and dynamic process family risk factors: Consequences for holistic adolescent functioning. *Journal of Marriage and Family, 69*, 654–675.

McWayne, C., Hampton, V., Fantuzzo, J., Cohen, H.L., & Sekino, Y. (2004). A multivariate examination of parent involvement and the social and academic competencies of urban kindergarten children. *Psychology in the Schools, 41*, 363–377.

Oates, G. L. St. C. (2009). An empirical test of five prominent explanations for the black-white performance gap. *Social Psychological Education, 12*, 415–441.

Park, N. (2011). Military children and families: Strengths and challenges during peace and war. *American Psychologist, 66*, 65–72. doi: 10.1037/a0021249

Parra, G.R., Dubois, D.L., & Sher, K.J. (2006). Investigation of profiles of risk factors for adolescent psychopathology: A person-centered approach. *Journal of Clinical Child and Adolescent Psychology, 35*, 386–402.

Ram, B., & Hou, F. (2003). Changes in family structure and child outcomes: Roles of economic and familial resources. *PSJ Policy Studies Journal, 31*, 309–330.

Raver, C. C., Gershoff, E. T., & Aber, J. L. (2007). Testing equivalence of mediating models of income, parenting, and school readiness for white, black, and Hispanic children in a national sample. *Child Development, 78*, 96–115.

Rogers, M. A., Theule, J., Ryan, B. A., Adams, G. R., & Keating, L. (2009). Parental involvement and children's school achievement evidence for mediating processes. *Canadian Journal of School Psychology, 24*, 34–57.

Simms, K. (2012). A hierarchical examination of the immigrant achievement gap: The additional power of nationality and educational selectivity over traditional explorations of race and socioeconomic status. *Journal of Advanced Academic, 23*, 72–98.

Smalls, C. (2009). African American adolescent engagement in the classroom and beyond: The roles of mother's racial socialization and democratic-involved parenting. *Journal of Youth and Adolescence, 38*, 204–213.

Smokowski, P.R., Mann, E.A., Reynolds, A.J., & Fraser, M.W. (2004). Childhood risk and protective factors and late adolescent adjustment in inner city minority youth. *Children and Youth Services Review, 26*, 63–91.

Somers, C. L., Chiodo, L. M., Yoon, J., Ratner, H., Barton, E., & Delaney-Black, V. (2011). Family disruption and academic functioning in urban, Black youth. *Psychology in the Schools, 48*, 357–370.

Stanton-Chapman, T. L., Chapman, D. A., Kaiser, A. P., & Hancock, T. B. (2004). Cumulative risk and low-income children's language development. *Topics in Early Childhood Special Education, 24*, 227–237.

Steinberg, L., Lamborn, S. D., Dornbusch, S. M., & Darling, N. (1992). Impact of parenting practices on adolescent achievement: Authoritative parenting, school involvement, and encouragement to succeed. *Child Development, 63*, 1266–1281.

Steinberg, L., Mounts, N. S., Lamborn, S. D., & Dornbusch, S. M. (1991). Authoritative parenting and adolescent adjustment across varied ecological niches. *Journal of Research on Adolescence, 1*, 19–36.

Van Dorn, R.A., Bowen, G.L., & Blau, J.R. (2006). The impact of community diversity and consolidated inequality on dropping out of high school. *Family Relations, 55*, 105–118.

Wang, M. T., & Huguley, J. P. (2012). Parental racial socialization as a moderator of the effects of racial discrimination on educational success among African American adolescent. *Child Development, 83*, 1716–1731.

White, K. R. (1982). The relation between socioeconomic status and academic achievement. *Psychological Bulletin, 91*, 461–481.

Zeiders, K., Roosa, M.W., & Tein, J.Y. (2011). Family structure and family processes in Mexican-American families. *Family Process, 50*, 77–91.

12

SCHOOL-BASED BULLYING: DEFINITION, PREVALENCE, ETIOLOGY, OUTCOMES, AND PREVENTIVE STRATEGIES

Dorothy L. Espelage and Cassandra L. Colbert

The U.S. Department of Education and the Centers for Disease Control and Prevention collaborated to develop a uniform research definition of bullying. This group defined bullying as follows: "Bullying is any unwanted aggressive behavior(s) by another youth or group of youths who are not siblings or current dating partners that involves an observed or perceived power imbalance and is repeated multiple times or is highly likely to be repeated. Bullying may inflict harm or distress on the targeted youth including physical, psychological, social, or educational harm" (Gladden, Vivolo-Kantor, Hamburger, & Lumpkin, 2014, p. 7). These behaviors include verbal and physical aggression that range in severity from making threats, spreading rumors, and social exclusion, to physical attacks causing injury. This definition emphasizes observable or non-observable aggressive behaviors, the (potentially) repetitive nature of these behaviors, and the imbalance of power between the individual/group perpetrator and victim. An imbalance of power exists when the perpetrator, or group of perpetrators, have more physical, social, or intellectual power than the victim. It is also important to define peer-victimization, which is used to refer to a form of peer abuse in which a child is frequently the target of peer aggression (Kochenderfer & Ladd, 1996). Therefore, bullying is a special case of peer-victimization, since the latter does not explicitly include the issues of power imbalance and intent included in the definition of bullying (Hunter, Boyle, & Warden, 2007).

It is critical for school staff and mental health professionals to take seriously even one bullying incident given the fact that targets of bullying often change their behaviors to prevent the recurrence (for review, see Espelage, 2015). For example, they might stop riding the bus, going to the lunchroom, and/or drop out of a sport or activity. In addition, school staff should ask the following questions of youth who experience bullying: (1) What is happening to you? (2) How long has it been going on? (3) Do you feel that you are able to defend, or protect, yourself? (4) Do you have anyone that you can talk to about the bullying? If they describe bullying that has been happening repeatedly, feelings of helplessness or vulnerability, and no one to talk to about the bullying, then the student should be given a suicide assessment and referred to counseling. This is extremely important as research has shown that there is an increased prevalence of depression and suicide ideation among both bullies and victims (Kaltiala-Heino, Rimpelä, Marttunen, Rimpelä, & Rantanen, 1999; Holt et al., 2015). Frequent exposure to victimization or bullying others has been related to high risks of depression, ideation, and suicide attempts compared with adolescents not involved in bullying behavior (Holt et al., 2015; Klomek, Marrocco, Kleinman, Schonfeld, & Gould, 2007). The fact that there are negative outcomes for both the victims and perpetrators demonstrates the need to create school environments where bullying is not tolerated.

Magnitude and Impact of Bullying Experiences

Bullying is a significant public health problem in the U.S. among school-aged youth. From 15% to 23% of elementary school students, and 20% to 28% of secondary school students, report being bullied within a six-month to one-year period (Carlyle & Steinman, 2007; National Center for Education Statistics, 2011; Turner, Finkelhor, Hamby, Shattuck, & Ormrod, 2011). Longitudinal data are quite clear that victims of bullying suffer in terms of their social and emotional outcomes (Ttofi, Farrington, Lösel, & Loeber, 2011) along with their physical health (Copeland et al., 2014). In a recent examination of a nationally representative study, early and late adolescents who perceived their perpetrator as having more power reported greater adverse outcomes (e.g., depression, suicidal ideation) than victims who did not perceive a power differential (Ybarra, Espelage, & Mitchell, 2014).

Not surprisingly, being bullied also has an impact on academic development and educational outcomes. Studies have documented that victims often experience depression, social anxiety, and low self-esteem, which could then contribute to academic challenges. Similar to the results with depression and suicidality, both bullies and bully-victims report academic, interpersonal, and intrapersonal challenges (Cook, Williams, Guerra, Kim, & Sadek, 2010). Bully-victims are individuals who perpetrate bullying behaviors and are also victimized. One study that looked at 3,530 elementary students found that victims and bully-victims were more likely to report feeling that they don't belong at school (Glew, Fan, Katon, Rivara, & Kernic, 2005). Another longitudinal study of 2,300 ethnically diverse sixth graders from 11 public middle schools showed that grade point averages and teacher-rated academic engagement were each predicted by both self-perceptions of victimization and peer nominations of victim reputation (Juvonen, Wang, & Espinoza (2010).

Several youth populations are at particular risk for being targeted by bullying and for directing bullying toward other students, including students with disabilities and gender non-conforming youth (Rose, Monda-Amaya, & Espelage, 2011, for review). A recent study of bully victimization among students with disabilities using the Special Education Elementary Longitudinal Study and the National Longitudinal Transition Study-2 longitudinal datasets revealed a prevalence rate of 24.5% in elementary school, 34.1% in middle school, and 26.6% in high school (Blake, Lund, Zhou, Kwok, & Benz, 2012). In a regional study of middle and high school youth (n = 21,646), students with disabilities were twice as likely to be identified as proactively engaging in bullying behavior and more likely to fight in a reactive manner than students without disabilities (Rose, Espelage, & Monda-Amaya, 2009). Rose and Espelage (2012) explored perpetration rates between students with emotional and behavioral disorders (EBD) and their peers without disabilities or with other disability labels (Other Health Impairment, Learning Disability, and Speech and Language Impairment). Results indicated that the students with EBD engaged in higher rates of proactive and reactive aggression perpetration than any other subgroup of students.

Research has consistently shown that sexual minority youth report high rates of peer victimization (Robinson & Espelage, 2011; 2012). The Gay, Lesbian, and Straight Education Network's (GLSEN) National Climate Study of 7,261 middle and high school students found that nearly 90% of lesbian, gay, bisexual, and transgender (LGBT) students experienced harassment at school in the past year; nearly 67% felt unsafe because of their sexual orientation; and nearly a third of LGBT students skipped at least one day of school in the past month because of safety concerns (Kosciw, Greytak, Diaz, & Bartkiewicz, 2010). Thus, it is clear that sexual minority youth are at greater risk for peer victimization than heterosexual youth. This difference has been theorized to be a result of prevailing homophobic beliefs and attitudes (Birkett & Espelage, 2015; Poteat & DiGiovanni, 2010). Thus, it is not the case that sexual identity or orientation contributes to the greater risk, but the fact that these students are growing up in environments that are homophobic and promote heteronormativity (Horn, Kosciw, & Russell, 2009).

Social-Ecological Framework

As defined and explained in the introduction of this book, a social-ecological model is useful in understanding school bullying and peer victimization as it focuses on how individual characteristics of children interact with environmental contexts, or systems, to promote or prevent victimization and perpetration (Espelage, 2012; Hong & Espelage, 2012).

Individual Characteristics

Socio-demographic characteristics, such as age, gender, and race/ethnicity, are frequently examined predictors of bullying behavior in school. Many studies report that boys in general are more likely to engage in bullying than girls (Espelage,

Low, Rao, Hong, & Little, 2014; Nansel et al., 2001). Despite this, other studies have failed to document significant sex differences in relational aggression or social forms of bullying (Card, Stuckey, Sawalani, & Little, 2008). Bullying is increasingly being viewed as a gendered set of behaviors where youth are targeted by either same- or other-sex peers in attempts to gain social status (Rodkin & Berger, 2008). Further, developmental trends indicate that bullying is a precursor to the use of homophobic epithets, which is in turn associated with sexual harassment during middle school (Espelage, Basile, & Hamburger, 2012; Espelage, Basile, De La Rue, & Hamburger, 2014) and with teen dating violence in high school (Espelage et al., 2014; Miller et al., 2013). Several studies have also looked at the role of race/ethnicity in bullying. In a nationally representative sample of grades 6 through 10 (*N*=7,182), African American adolescents were involved in more bullying (physical, verbal, or cyber) but less victimization; verbal or relational (Wang, Iannotti, & Nansel, 2009). In another study of 11,033 adolescents, also in grades 6 through 10, Black adolescents reported a significantly lower prevalence of victimization than White and Hispanic students (Spriggs, Iannotti, Nansel, & Haynie, 2007). Furthermore, although school satisfaction and performance were negatively associated with bullying involvement for White and Hispanic students, school factors were largely unrelated to bullying among Black students (Spriggs et al., 2007). One needs to be careful of making any definitive conclusions about race and ethnicity with bullying as several other factors come into play. Lastly, numerous studies have shown that bullying behaviors peak during the middle school years and then gradually decline; however, they can lead to sexual harassment and teen dating violence, as mentioned above (Espelage et al., 2014; Miller et al., 2013).

Family Characteristics

Youth who bully tend to have parents who do not provide adequate supervision or are not actively involved in the lives of their children (Espelage, Bosworth, & Simon, 2000; Georgiou & Fanti, 2010). In other instances, parents may encourage the use of aggressive and retaliatory behaviors (Smokowski & Kopasz, 2005). In a recent longitudinal study, exposure to family conflict (sibling aggression, yelling) was associated with greater bully perpetration for a large sample of middle school students (Espelage et al., 2014). Further, children who are victims of bullying more often come from abusive families or inconsistent parenting (Georgiou & Fanti, 2010). Supportive familial relations can also buffer the impact of involvement with bully experiences. When victims of bullying have warm relationships with their families, they have more positive outcomes, both emotionally and behaviorally (Holt & Espelage, 2007). These positive parent-child interactions provide children with the opportunity to talk about their bullying experiences and can provide guidance on how to cope with these events.

Peers

Bullying and peer victimization rarely takes place in isolated dyadic interactions, but instead often occurs in the presence of other students. Youth who have friends that bully will bully more over time (Espelage, Holt, & Henkel, 2003) and those who have friends who engage in homophobic name-calling will use this language (Birkett & Espelage, 2015). In a comprehensive meta-analysis, Cook and colleagues (2010) found that youth in middle school who bullied other students had greater social status among peers, whereas younger children who bullied were socially rejected. Further, students may promote bullying by actively joining in or passively accepting bullying behaviors, or conversely reduce bullying incidents by intervening to stop bullying or by defending the victim (Espelage, Green, & Polanin, 2012).

Interactions Among Microsystems

In this chapter, we will look at only a couple of the key microsystems when understanding school-based bullying: 1) the interaction between students, teachers, and administrators; and 2) genes and classroom norms.

Interactions among microsystems: Students, teachers, and administrators. Research indicates that relations among students, teachers, and administrators matter. Troop-Gordon and Ladd (2015) highlighted an inherent disconnect in the bully prevention field with their statement, "Although teachers are often called upon to reduce children's bullying and aggression, little is known regarding teachers' responses to students' harassment of peers or the beliefs which may inform their response strategies." Indeed, a PsycINFO® search with the key words "teachers" and "bully prevention" yields 33 scholarly articles, modest in comparison to the over 1,000 articles published on bullying. This disconnect between basic research and prevention practices in relation to teachers is further exacerbated when teachers are often the individuals who are delivering classroom-based bully prevention curriculum (for review of programs, see Espelage, 2015). The trend from having outside practitioners, or school counselors, implement curriculum to teacher implementers suggests that we need to know more about how teacher attitudes, behaviors, and practices might impede or foster prevention efforts.

Many national websites on bully prevention provide concrete steps on how teachers should respond to bullying (see resources); however, the evidence for many of these suggestions is lacking and it is not clear which strategies actually lead to reductions in peer victimization. Troop-Gordon and Ladd (2015) addressed the gap in the literature by examining the short-term longitudinal relations between teachers' beliefs and responses to peer victimization and how these beliefs and responses relate to students' aggressive behavior and victimization among 170 6th- and 7th-grade teachers and 2,938 of their students. Several novel findings were found. First, gender of the victim makes a difference in how teachers respond. Teachers contacted parents and separated students more for boys than girls; however, they were more likely to tell girls than boys to work out the problem on their own, to assert themselves, and avoid aggressive peers. Second, when teachers held beliefs that peer victimization is normative, they were more likely to tell children to work it out and less likely to reprimand the aggressor. Interestingly, when teachers advocated for the victim to take an assertive approach, this was associated with higher levels of aggression and victimization concurrently, but not over the course of the year. Third, like previous research with younger students (Kochenderfer-Ladd & Pelletier, 2008), when teachers separated students in response to aggression, this was associated with lower levels of aggression, declines in classroom-level peer victimization, and declines in aggression for highly aggressive girls. These findings suggest that there are simple strategies that teachers can use to prevent victimization, which is helpful at a time when teachers are asked to address bullying through curriculum in a climate of high-stakes testing, heightened teacher accountability, and diminishing resources. Much of this scholarship is predicated on the assumptions that teachers would either witness the victimization or students would report it; however, often teachers do not witness these events and students do not report them. We do know that when students do tell adults or teachers do observe a situation, they are more likely to respond effectively if they feel highly prepared to handle bullying situations (Novick & Isaacs, 2010). Thus, it is imperative that pre-service teacher training programs include bully prevention and concrete strategies in the curriculum, as suggested by Troop-Gordon and Ladd (2015). Unfortunately, there is not a program that has been developed and rigorously evaluated, which results in teacher training programs varying in the way this is incorporated into the curriculum.

Oldenburg and colleagues (2015) expanded on the literature on teacher characteristics to include attributions that teachers make about why bullying occurs, including internal (e.g., student fault) and external (e.g., due to things out of control of the student); their own bullying and victimization experiences; and their teaching experience. Further, these authors examined the association between multiple grade classrooms as predictors of classroom-level victimization. External attributions were associated with more victimization, and closer examination of the items assessing external attributions reveals that these items really demonstrate that teachers are *blaming* students and their families for the bullying. This finding parallels the research among youth showing that peers would defend a victim when they had empathy for the victim (Espelage et al., 2012; Gini, Albiero, Benelli, & Altoe, 2007) and felt a personal responsibility to intervene (Poyhonen, Juvonen, & Salmivalli, 2010). Surprising to Oldenburg and colleagues, teachers' self-perceived ability to handle bullying was not related to classroom victimization, although it was reported as marginally significant ($p < .08$). This finding could be attributed to the tendency for teachers to endorse "neutral" responses about their ability to manage bullying. It would be important to extend this work to include more data from the students about how their teachers handle bullying.

Serdiouk, Rodkin, Madill, Logis, and Gest (2015) also examined classroom characteristics on peer victimization rates. They extended this work to the relations among classroom peer ecologies, teacher practices, rejection, and peer victimization over one year among 1020 elementary teachers from 54 classrooms. Results indicated that classrooms where victimized youth were more centralized, and there was greater rejection, led to evident increases in victimization over the school year; in contrast, when teachers reported making efforts to equalize social status, there was less victimization. Teacher attunement to victimization of students and strategies to prevent aggression by the teachers did not mitigate the rejection-victimization connection, leading Serdiouk et al. (2015) to argue for the focus of interventions on classroom level victimization, rejection, and teacher's management of social status. Indeed, as teachers are often described as the "invisible hand" (Farmer, Lines, & Hamm, 2011), they are instrumental in creating classrooms with fewer rejected and victimized youth. However, making teachers aware of the pivotal role that they play in creating safe and inclusive classrooms may require training as opposed to being something that is organic to teachers. For example, Hamm, Farmer, Dadisman, Gravelle, and Murray (2011) found that where teachers and students agreed on the social dynamics in the classroom, there was positive improvement in students' perceptions of the school environment.

Finally, in a recent multi-level study of 3,600 students across 36 middle schools, less bullying, physical fighting, victimization, and greater willingness to intervene were reported in schools where staff reported that they felt supported by their administration to address bullying in their classrooms and schools (Espelage, Polanin, & Low, 2014).

Interactions among microsystems: Genes & classroom norms. Expression of genetic predispositions for aggression in classroom settings appears to be dependent on the classroom norms around aggression. Brendgen, Girard, Vitaro, Dionne, and Boivin (2014) represents prevention science research that pushes the aggression and peer victimization field into more serious conversations about the interaction of genes and the school classroom environment. Data from 197 monozygotic and dizygotic twin pairs in the 4th grade found that youth with a genetic disposition for aggressive behavior display those behaviors only in classrooms where classroom norms are favorable to aggression. Further, Brendgen et al.'s (2014) findings provide some evidence of how bullies occupy "two social worlds" (Farmer et al., 2010). Some youth are social integrated and some are marginalized. Indeed, classroom norms that do not support aggression are more likely to produce victimized youth, possibly contributing to social marginalization, whereas social integrated youth in classrooms with norms supportive of aggression are less at-risk to be victimized (Farmer et al., 2010). The finding that some aggressive youth are well-integrated into their peer culture is not a new finding; the research pioneer Professor Daniel Olweus (1978) has written about these youth for over three decades. In summary, the research suggests that no youth is destined to be aggressive in all contexts, but rather the environmental conditions dictate the extent to which their genetic disposition for aggressive behavior is enacted.

School-based Bully Prevention Approaches

Almost every state in the United States requires some type of bully prevention policy and/or intervention. Thus, bully prevention programs are being evaluated to determine their efficacy to reduce bullying and peer victimization. Overall, these programs differ in their efficacy across contexts (Ttofi & Farrington, 2011) or have produced mixed results (Pearce, Cross, Monks, Waters, & Falconer, 2011). The most comprehensive meta-analysis included a review of 44 rigorous program evaluations and randomized clinical trials (RCT; Ttofi & Farrington, 2011). Ttofi and Farrington (2011) found that the programs, on average, were associated with a 20%–23% decrease in bullying perpetration and a 17%–20% decrease in victimization (Ttofi & Farrington, 2011).

Ttofi and Farrington (2011) found a few program elements that appear to be driving these reductions. Decreases in rates of *victimization* were associated with the following special program elements: disciplinary (non-punitive) methods, parent training/meetings, use of videos, and cooperative group work. In addition, the duration and intensity of the program for children and teachers were significantly associated with a decrease in victimization. Interestingly, more than just these factors were needed to bring about changes in bully perpetration. Specific program elements that were associated with decreases in rates of *bully perpetration* included: parent training/meetings, improved playground supervision, disciplinary (non-punitive) methods, classroom management, teacher training, classroom rules, whole-school anti-bullying policy, school conferences, information for parents (ranging from information in newsletters to suggestions for helping children with bullying situations), and cooperative group work. Further, the number of elements and the duration and intensity of the program for teachers and children were significantly associated with a decrease in bullying in studies in Norway and Europe. Given the time and resource demands associated with this comprehensive approach, it has been difficult to implement programs that meet all of these elements in the United States. While schools recognize the need for bullying prevention efforts, costs, training, academic priorities, and other factors are often barriers for ideal implementation and ongoing management of such programs. In addition, there is a significant need to methodically investigate the programs that do exist for their effectiveness as it related to social, emotional, and academic outcomes.

Social-Emotional Learning Programs

Ttofi and Farrington (2011) found that across the 44 studies on bullying prevention programs, use of a curriculum was the second most frequent program element ($n = 34$), but this element was not significantly associated with decreases in bully perpetration or victimization (Ttofi & Farrington, 2011). However, the majority of these programs are narrowly focused on the topic of bullying, and do not address the numerous risk and protective factors that predict bullying and victimization (Espelage, 2015). In contrast, social-emotional learning programs to address bullying and other forms of aggression draw from the risk and protective framework literature and purposively teach a wide range of skills to prevent conflicts and skills to prevent escalation of conflicts (e.g., communication, problem-solving, emotion regulation). Indeed, school-based social-emotional (SEL) programs that address interpersonal conflict and teach emotion management have succeeded in reducing youth violence, including bullying, fighting, and disruptive behaviors in classrooms (Espelage, Low, Polanin, & Brown, 2013; Wilson & Lipsey, 2007). Although additional research is needed, social-emotional learning programs offer a good foundation for schools in order to teach students a variety of helpful skills and to possibly mitigate bullying and peer victimization.

Take-Home Points

- Bullying is a public health issue that needs to be addressed immediately and through systematic school-wide policies, reporting, investigation, and follow through.
- Bullying is a form of aggression that involves a power dynamic, is intentional, and is often repeated (do not wait for it to happen more than once, however, before responding).
- Students with disabilities and gender non-conforming youth report high rates of victimization.
- Bullying involvement as a perpetrator and/or victim is best understood as being predicted by individual, family, peer, and school-related variables.
- Interaction among teachers, students, and the classroom environment has a significant impact on whether bullying and victimization will occur.
- Efficacy of bully prevention programs is lower in the U.S. than other countries, but research on social-emotional learning programs in the U.S. is showing favorable results in reducing bullying, fighting, and other disruptive behavior.

Resources

- http://www.aauw.org
- http://www.cdc.gov/violenceprevention/youthviolence/bullyingresearch/
- http://www.cfchildren.org/bullying-prevention
- http://www.ed.gov/category/keyword/bullying
- http://www.glsen.org/cgi-bin/iowa/all/home/index.html
- http://www.stopbullying.gov/respond/index.html

References

Birkett, M., & Espelage, D.L. (2015). Homophobic name-calling, peer-groups, and masculinity: The socialization of homophobic behavior in adolescents. *Social Development, 24*(1), 184–205.

Blake, J.J., Lund, E.M., Zhou, Q., Kwok, O., & Benz, M.R. (2012). National prevalence rates of bully victimization among students with disabilities in the United States. *School Psychology Quarterly, 27*, 210–222.

Brendgen, M., Girard, A., Vitaro, F., Dionne, G., & Boivin, M. (2014). The dark side of friends: A genetically informed study of victimization within early adolescents' friendships. *Journal of Clinical Child & Adolescent Psychology*. doi: 10.1080/15374416.2013.873984

Card, N., Stuckey, B., Sawalani, G., & Little, T. (2008). Direct and indirect aggression during childhood and adolescence: A meta-analytic review of gender differences, intercorrelations, and relations to maladjustment. *Child Development, 79*(5), 1185–1229.

Carlyle, K.E., & Steinman, K.J. (2007). Demographic differences in the prevalence, co-occurrence, and correlates of adolescent bullying at school. *Journal of School Health*, 77(9), 623–629.

Cook, C.R., Williams, K.R., Guerra, N.G., Kim, T.E., & Sadek, S. (2010). Predictors of bullying and victimization in childhood and adolescence: A meta-analytic investigation. *School Psychology Quarterly, 25*, 65–83.

Copeland, W.E., Wolke, D., Lereya, S.T., Shanahan, L., Worthman, C., & Costello, E.J. (2014). Childhood bullying involvement predicts low-grade systemic inflammation into adulthood. *Proceedings of the National Academy of Sciences, 111*, 7570–7575.

Espelage, D.L. (2012). Bullying prevention: A research dialogue with Dorothy Espelage. *Prevention Researcher, 19*(3), 17–19.

Espelage, D.L. (2015). Emerging issues in school bullying research & prevention science. In E.T. Emme & E. Sabornie (Eds.), *Handbook of classroom management: Research, practice, and contemporary issues*. New York: Taylor & Francis.

Espelage, D.L., Basile, K.C., De La Rue, L., & Hamburger, M. (2014). Longitudinal associations among bully, homophobic teasing and sexual violence perpetration among middle school students. *Journal of Interpersonal Violence*. Online first.

Espelage, D.L., Basile, K.C., & Hamburger, M.E. (2012). Bullying experiences and co-occurring sexual violence perpetration among middle school students: Shared and unique risk factors. *Journal of Adolescent Health, 50*, 60–65.

Espelage, D.L., Bosworth, K., & Simon, T.R. (2000). Examining the social context of bullying behaviors in early adolescence. *Journal of Counseling and Development, 78*, 326–333.

Espelage, D.L., Green, H.D., & Polanin, J. (2012). Willingness to intervene in bullying episodes among middle school students: individual and peer-group influences. *Journal of Early Adolescence, 32*, 776–801.

Espelage, D.L., Holt, M.K., & Henkel, R.R. (2003). Examination of peer-group contextual effects on aggression during early adolescence. *Child Development, 74*, 205–220.

Espelage, D.L., Low, S., Polanin, J., & Brown, E. (2013). The impact of a middle-school program to reduce aggression, victimization, and sexual violence. *Journal of Adolescent Health, 53*(2), 180–186.

Espelage, D.L., Low, S., Rao, M.A., Hong, J.S. & Little, T.D. (2014). Family violence, bullying, fighting, and substance use among adolescents: a longitudinal mediational model. *Journal of Research on Adolescence, 24*, 337–349.

Espelage, D.L., Polanin, J., & Low, S. (2014). Teacher & staff perceptions of school environment as predictors of student aggression, victimization, and willingness to intervene in bullying situations. *School Psychology Quarterly, 29*(3), 287–305.

Farmer, T.W., Lines, M.M., & Hamm, J.V. (2011). Revealing the invisible hand: The role of teachers in children's peer experiences. *Journal of Applied Developmental Psychology, 32*, 247–256.

Farmer, T.W., Petrin, R.A., Robertson, D.L., Fraser, M.W., Hall, C.M., Day. S.H., & Dadisman, K. (2010). Peer relations of bullies, bully-victims, and victims: The two social worlds of bullying in second-grade classrooms. *Elementary School Journal, 110*, 364–392.

Georgiou, S.N., & Fanti, K.A. (2010). A transactional model of bullying and victimization. *Social Psychology of Education, 13*(3), 295–311.

Gini, G., Albiero, P., Benelli, & Altoe, G. (2007). Does empathy predict adolescents' bullying and defending behavior? *Aggressive Behavior, 33*, 467–476.

Gladden, R.M., Vivolo-Kantor, A.M., Hamburger, M.E., & Lumpkin, C.D. (2014). *Bullying surveillance among youths: Uniform definitions for public health and recommended data elements, Version 1.0*. Atlanta, GA; National Centers for Injury Prevention and Control, Centers for Disease Control and Prevention and U.S. Department of Education.

Glew, G.M., Fan, M.Y., Katon, W., Rivara, F.P., & Kernic, M.A. (2005). Bullying, psychosocial adjustment, and academic performance in elementary school. *Archives of Pediatrics & Adolescent Medicine, 159*(11), 1026–1031.

Hamm, J.V., Farmer, T W., Dadisman, K., Gravelle, M., & Murray, A.R. (2011). Teachers' attunement to students' peer group affiliations as a source of improved student experiences of the school social-affective context following the middle school transition. *Journal of Applied Developmental Psychology, 32*, 267–277.

Holt, M.K., & Espelage, D.L. (2007). Perceived social support among bullies, victims, and bully-victims. *Journal of Youth and Adolescence, 36*(6), 984–994.

Holt, M.K., Vivolo-Kantor, A.M., Polanin, J.R., Holland, K.M., DeGue, S., Matiasko, J.L., . . . Reid, G.R. (2015). Bullying and suicidal ideation and behaviors: A meta-analysis. *Pediatrics, 135*, e496–e509.

Hong, J.S., & Espelage, D.L. (2012). A review of research on bullying and peer victimization in school: An ecological system analysis. *Aggression and Violent Behavior, 17*, 311–322.

Horn, S.S., Kosciw, J.G., & Russell, S.T. (2009). Special issue introduction: New research on lesbian, gay, bisexual, and transgender youth: Studying lives in context. *Journal of Youth and Adolescence, 38*, 863–866.

Hunter, S.C., Boyle, J.M., & Warden, D. (2007). Perceptions and correlates of peer-victimization and bullying. *British Journal of Educational Psychology, 77*(4), 797–810.

Juvonen, J., Wang, Y., & Espinoza, G. (2010). Bullying experiences and compromised academic performance across middle school grades. *The Journal of Early Adolescence, 31*(1), 152–173.

Kaltiala-Heino, R., Rimpelä, M., Marttunen, M., Rimpelä, A., & Rantanen, P. (1999). Bullying, depression, and suicidal ideation in Finnish adolescents: school survey. *BMJ, 319*(7206), 348–351.

Klomek, A.B., Marrocco, F., Kleinman, M., Schonfeld, I.S., & Gould, M.S. (2007). Bullying, depression, and suicidality in adolescents. *Journal of the American Academy of Child & Adolescent Psychiatry, 46*(1), 40–49.

Kochenderfer, B.J., & Ladd, G.W. (1996). Peer victimization: Cause or consequence of school maladjustment? *Child Development, 67*(4), 1305–1317.

Kochenderfer-Ladd, B., & Pelletier, M.E. (2008) Teachers' views and beliefs about bullying: Influences on classroom management strategies and students' coping with peer victimization. *Journal of School Psychology, 46*, 431–453.

Kosciw, J.G., Greytak, E.A., Diaz, E.M., & Bartkiewicz, M.J. (2010). *The 2009 National School Climate Survey: The experiences of lesbian, gay, bisexual and transgender youth in our nation's schools*. New York: Gay, Lesbian, and Straight Education Network.

Low, S., & Espelage, D.L. (2014). Conduits from community violence exposure to peer aggression and victimization: Contributions of parental monitoring, impulsivity and deviancy. *Journal of Counseling Psychology, 61*, 221–231.

Miller, S., Williams, J., Cutbush, S., Gibbs, D., Clinton-Sherrod, M., & Jones, S. (2013). Dating violence, bullying, and sexual harassment: Longitudinal profiles and transitions over time. *Journal of Youth and Adolescence, 42*(4), 607–618.

Nansel, T.R., Overpeck, M., Pilla, R.S., Ruan, W.J., Simons-Morton, B., & Scheidt, P. (2001). Bullying behaviors among US youth: Prevalence and association with psychosocial adjustment. *The Journal of the American Medical Association, 285*, 2094–2100.

National Center for Education Statistics. (2011). *Achievement gaps: How Hispanic and White students in public schools perform in mathematics and reading on the National Assessment of Educational Progress*. Statistical Analysis Report. NCES 2011–459.

Novick, R.M., & Isaacs, J. (2010). Telling is compelling: The impact of student reports of bullying on teacher intervention. *Educational Psychology, 30*(3), 283–296.

Oldenburg, B., van Duijn, M., Sentse, M., Huitsing, G., van der Ploeg, R., Salmivalli, C., & Veenstra, R. (2015). Teacher characteristics and peer victimization in elementary schools: A classroom-level perspective. *Journal of Abnormal Child Psychology, 43*(1), 33–44.

Olweus, D. (1978). *Aggression in school: Bullies and whipping boys*. Washington: Hemisphere.

Pearce, N., Cross, D., Monks, H., Waters, S., & Falconer, S. (2011). Current evidence of best practice in whole-school bullying intervention and its potential to inform cyberbullying interventions. *Australian Journal of Guidance and Counselling, 21*(1), 1–21.

Poteat, P.V., & DiGiovanni, C.D. (2010). When biased language use is associated with bullying and dominance behavior: The moderating effect of prejudice. *Journal of Youth and Adolescence, 39*, 1123–1133.

Pozzoli, T., & Gini, G. (2010). Active defending and passive bystanding behavior in bullying: The role of personal characteristics and perceived pressure. *Journal of Abnormal Child Psychology, 38*, 815–827.

Poyhonen, V., Juvonen, J., & Salmivalli, C. (2010). What does it take to stand up for the victim of bullying? The interplay between personal and social factors. *Merrill-Palmer Quarterly, 56*(2), 143–163.

Robinson, J.P., & Espelage, D.L. (2011). Inequities in educational and psychological outcomes between LGBTQ and straight students in middle and high school. *Educational Researcher, 40*(7), 315–330.

Robinson, J.P., & Espelage, D.L. (2012). Bullying explains only part of LGBTQ–heterosexual risk disparities implications for policy and practice. *Educational Researcher, 41*(8), 309–319.

Rodkin, P.C., & Berger, C. (2008). Who bullies whom? Social status asymmetries by victim gender. *International Journal of Behavioral Development, 32*, 473–485.

Rose, C.A., Espelage, D.L., & Monda-Amaya, L.E. (2009). Bullying and victimisation rates among students in general and special education: A comparative analysis. *Educational Psychology, 29*(7), 761–776.

Rose, C.A., Monda-Amaya, L.E., & Espelage, D.L. (2011). Bullying perpetration and victimization in special education: A review of the literature. *Remedial and Special Education, 32*, 114–130.

Serdiouk, M., Rodkin, P., Madill, R., Logis, H., & Gest, S. (2015). Rejection and victimization among elementary school children: The buffering role of classroom-level predictors. *Journal of Abnormal Child Psychology, 43*(1), 5–17.

Smokowski, P.R., & Kopasz, K.H. (2005). Bullying in school: An overview of types, effects, family characteristics, and intervention strategies. *Children & Schools, 27*(2), 101–110.

Spriggs, A.L., Iannotti, R.J., Nansel, T.R., & Haynie, D.L. (2007). Adolescent bullying involvement and perceived family, peer and school relations: Commonalities and differences across race/ethnicity. *Journal of Adolescent Health*, *41*(3), 283–293.

Troop-Gordon, W., & Ladd, G.W. (2015). Teachers' victimization-related beliefs and strategies: Associations with students' aggressive behavior and peer victimization. *Journal of Abnormal Child Psychology*, *43*(1), 45–60.

Ttofi, M.M., & Farrington, D.P. (2011). Effectiveness of school-based programs to reduce bullying: A systematic and meta-analytic review. *Journal of Experimental Criminology*, *7*, 27–56.

Ttofi, M.M., Farrington, D.P., Lösel, F., Loeber, R. (2011). Do the victims of school bullies tend to become depressed later in life? A systematic review and meta-analysis of longitudinal studies. *Journal of Aggression, Conflict and Peace Research*, *3*(2), 63–73.

Turner, H.A., Finkelhor, D., Hamby, S.L., Shattuck, A., & Ormrod, R.K. (2011). Specifying type and location of peer victimization in a national sample of children and youth. *Journal of Youth and Adolescence*, *40*(8), 1052–1067.

Wang, J., Iannotti, R.J., & Nansel, T.R. (2009). School bullying among adolescents in the United States: Physical, verbal, relational, and cyber. *Journal of Adolescent Health*, *45*(4), 368–375.

Wilson, S.J., & Lipsey, M.W. (2007). School-based interventions for aggressive and disruptive behavior: Update of a meta-analysis. *American Journal of Preventive Medicine*, *33*, S130–S143.

Ybarra, M., Espelage, D.L., & Mitchell, K.J. (2014). Differentiating youth who are bullied from other victims of peer-aggression: the importance of differential power and repetition. *Journal of Adolescent Health*. Online first.

13

INTERPERSONAL VIOLENCE (DATING AND SEXUAL VIOLENCE)

Andra Teten Tharp

Dating and sexual violence are prevalent issues among middle and high school youth. Experiencing violence is associated with a variety of negative health consequences, in addition to poor academic performance and re-victimization in college. Adolescents may be at risk for perpetrating dating and sexual violence as a result of a variety of factors, including their attitudes and behaviors, past experiences, family factors, and peer group. Middle and high school are key times to implement dating and sexual violence prevention that address these risk factors and build healthy relationships. A variety of evidence-based strategies are available that can be implemented during the school day, afterschool by coaches, in the community, and with families. Towards this end and in order to equip schools and communities with the information needed to address dating and sexual violence, the current chapter summarizes the best available research evidence on the prevalence of dating and sexual violence, risk and protective factors for perpetration, commonly used measures assessing violence among adolescents, effective programs, and emerging approaches for adolescents. Dating and sexual violence are preventable, and multiple approaches exist that can be used to support healthy and safe youth relationships.

Understanding Dating and Sexual Violence

Dating violence is any psychological/emotional, physical, or sexual violence perpetrated by one partner towards a current or former dating partner; violence can

---

Author's Note: The findings and conclusions in this report are those of the authors and do not necessarily represent the official position of the Centers for Disease Control and Prevention. Andra Teten Tharp is now with the Air Force Sexual Assault Prevention and Response Office.

occur in opposite-sex or same-sex relationships and may take place in person or electronically (Centers for Disease Control and Prevention, 2014). Dating among adolescents is amorphous (Teten, Ball, Valle, Noonan, & Rosenbluth, 2009); may be short-term, long-term, monogamous, non-monogamous, dyadic or group-based; and may or may not include sexual intimacy. Dating violence can occur in any of these dating contexts. Sexual violence is sexual activity where consent is not obtained or freely given, including when the victim is unable to consent or refuses (Basile, Smith, Breiding, Black, & Mahendra, 2015). A range of behaviors from unwanted touching to forced penetration are considered to be sexually violent. Sexual violence can be perpetrated by anyone, such as a dating partner, stranger, acquaintance, authority figure, or family member (Basile et al., 2015).

Unfortunately, many adolescents experience dating and sexual violence. For example, the 2013 Youth Risk Behavior Survey (YRBS) indicates that among the 73.9% of high school youth who had been on a date in the 12 months prior to the survey, approximately 10.3% (13.0% girls, 7.4% boys) reported physical dating violence victimization, and 10.4% (14.4% girls, 6.2% boys) reported sexual dating violence victimization in the 12 months prior to the survey. Among all youth surveyed, 7.3% (10.5% girls, 4.2% boys) reported forced intercourse by anyone at some point in their lives (Kann et al., 2014). When psychological, physical, and sexual dating violence are measured, up to 30% of youth report dating violence victimization across studies (Teten et al., 2009). The 2011 National Intimate Partner and Sexual Violence Survey found that among adults who experienced intimate partner violence, the adult form of dating violence, 22% of women and 15% of men first experienced this kind of violence between ages 11 and 17 (Breiding, Chen, & Black, 2014). Moreover, physical dating violence increases in prevalence through high school and appears to peak at approximately ages 17–18 (O'Leary & Slep, 2012), making middle and high school critical times for violence prevention and intervention.

Some young people are more likely than others to experience dating violence. Although men and women often report comparable frequencies of some physically violent acts (Archer, 2002), women and girls are more likely than boys to experience severe physical violence and sexual violence, making them particularly at risk for these types of violence (Black et al., 2011; Teten et al., 2009). Sexual minority youth report significantly higher rates of physical dating violence than heterosexual youth. Using data from local YRBS surveys conducted between 2001 and 2011, Luo, Stone, and Teten Tharp (2014) found 10.7% of heterosexual youth compared to 21.5% of bisexual youth and 24.6% of lesbian/gay youth reported experiencing physical dating violence victimization in the 12 months prior to the survey. The reasons why these groups are at higher risk for victimization are not well understood, though a variety of hypotheses have been developed (see Chapter 10, "Mental Health Concerns Among LGBTQ Youth in Schools"). Nonetheless, it is critical that these findings do not translate to victim blaming, but instead that young people who experience victimization have access to services and that potential perpetrators are exposed to effective prevention and intervention programs.

Dating and sexual violence have been associated with a variety of negative consequences. Longitudinal studies have shown that experiencing dating violence is associated with symptoms of depression and anxiety, substance use, antisocial behavior, suicidal ideation, and re-victimization during college (CDC, 2014). Cross-sectional studies have found direct associations between physical dating violence victimization and school attachment, and indirect associations between physical dating violence victimization and thoughts of dropping out of school and poor grades mediated by mental health issues, such as depression and substance use (Banyard & Cross, 2008). Similarly, sexual violence has been associated with suicidal ideation and substance use (Basile et al., 2006), as well as pregnancy (Holmes, Resnick, Kilpatrick, & Best, 1996) and other physical health issues such as chronic pelvic pain (Jewkes, Sen, Garcia-Moreno, 2002) among women. Dating and sexual violence may directly affect academic performance or performance could be negatively affected by the results of violence, such as injury and pregnancy, thus underscoring the need for prevention and intervention.

Although risk factors do not guarantee that an individual will perpetrate violence and protective factors do not guarantee that they will not, identifying risk and protective factors for dating and sexual violence is critical in order to understand which individuals and groups are at-risk for violence and to design effective prevention programs that address these factors. Table 13.1 provides a summary of the risk and protective factors for perpetration of dating and sexual violence based

TABLE 13.1 Risk and Protective Factors for Sexual Violence and Dating Violence Perpetration

Factor Category	*Sexual Violence (SV) Perpetration*** *(Teten Tharp, DeGue et al., 2013)*	*Dating Violence (DV) Perpetration (Vagi et al., 2013)*
Individual Level		
Violence-Related Cognitions	Acceptance of violence Dominance Competitiveness	Aggression-tolerant attitudes Acceptance of violence in dating relationships Emotional distress
Violence-Related Behaviors	Aggression Prior suicidal behavior	Fighting Antisocial behavior Violent behavior History of sexual, verbal, and/or physical aggression Prior dating violence Past suicide attempt Use of aggressive media

(*Continued*)

TABLE 13.1 (Continued)

Factor Category	*Sexual Violence (SV) Perpetration** (Teten Tharp, DeGue et al., 2013)*	*Dating Violence (DV) Perpetration (Vagi et al., 2013)*
Sex-related Thoughts/ Behaviors	Sexual fantasies Willingness to commit SV Victim blame Multiple sexual partners Impersonal sex Early initiation of sex Sexual risk taking Motivation for sex/sex drive SV victimization in adolescence/ adulthood Past SV perpetration Exposure to sexually explicit media Perpetrator positive for sexually transmitted infection Cue misinterpretation	Sexually active in middle school Desiring to have sex with dating partner High number of sex partners Having sex before love-telling
Substance Use	Alcohol use*	Alcohol use Marijuana use Other drug use
Gender-based Cognitions	Rape myth acceptance Hostility towards women Traditional gender role adherence Hypermasculinity	
Mental Health Issues		Depression Anxiety Trauma-related anger Trauma symptoms
Protective Factors	Empathy Emotional health ** Connectedness** Academic achievement***	Empathy Believing dating violence is wrong High grade point average High verbal IQ
Family		
Exposure to Violence	Child sexual abuse Child physical abuse Child emotional abuse Child maltreatment* Exposure to parental violence/ family context	Childhood physical abuse Parental marital conflict Intrafamilial violence Parental physical punishment (Low) Father-child hostility Harsh parenting practices

Factor Category	*Sexual Violence (SV) Perpetration** (Teten Tharp, DeGue et al., 2013)*	*Dating Violence (DV) Perpetration (Vagi et al., 2013)*
Poor Family Relationship Quality	Parent-child relationship quality*	Negative parent-child interactions Aversive family communication
Poor Parenting Skills		Unskilled parenting Low parental monitoring Parent-child boundary violations
Protective Factors	Parents' use of reasoning to resolve conflict**	Positive relationship with mother
Peer		
Peer Attitudes/ Behaviors	Peer approval for forced sex Peer pressure for sexual activity Peer sexual aggression	Friends who are perpetrators and/or victims of DV Involvement with antisocial peers Low friendship quality Hostile friendships Engagement in peer violence
Association with Hypermasculine or Deviant Peer Groups	Fraternity membership Sports participation Gang membership	
Intimate relationships		
Partner Relationship Quality	Relationship conflict/partner violence	Hostile/Conflict couple relationship Partner's use of physical aggression
Intimate Partner Processes	Relationship processes Casual relationship status	
Community		
Protective Factors		School attachment

**Studies* supporting this factor involved adult samples.
***Effect* found for male participants only
****Effect* found for female participants only
Note. Different methods were used in Teten Tharp, DeGue et al. (2013) and Vagi et al. (2013), such that risk and protective factors for sexual violence may have been drawn from cross-sectional or longitudinal studies, whereas risk and protective factors for dating violence were drawn only from longitudinal studies. Teten Tharp, DeGue et al. (2013) reviewed studies of adolescent and adult perpetrators, whereas Vagi et al. (2013) reviewed studies of adolescents and young adults.

on results from two recent reviews (Teten Tharp, DeGue et al., 2013; Vagi et al., 2013). As demonstrated in the table, multiple domains of risk exist for each form of violence, including substance use, sexual risk behaviors, youth violence, and attitudes supporting violence. Moreover, family and peer groups are also important considerations for risk, in that witnessing or experiencing violence in the home or having friends who support the use of violence or engage in relationship violence increases one's risk for perpetration. School-related factors can also serve as protective factors; for example, academic achievement was protective for high school girls' perpetration of sexual violence (Borowsky, Hogan & Ireland, 1997) and high grade point average and verbal IQ have been associated with lower levels of dating violence perpetration (Cleveland, Herrera, & Stuewig, 2003). Importantly, this work suggests that multiple factors exist across contexts, relationships, and development. Therefore, effective prevention and intervention strategies must also take into account the multiple domains of risk.

Common Measures of Dating and Sexual Violence Used Among Adolescents

A variety of measures have been used to assess dating and sexual violence, although three primary measures of dating violence among adolescents are used (Smith et al., in press): The Safe Dates Psychological and Physical Dating Abuse Scale (Foshee et al., 1996; 94 items); the Revised Conflict Tactics Scale (CTS-2, Straus, Hamby, Boney-McCoy, & Sugarman, 1996; 78 items); and Conflict in Adolescent Dating Relationships Inventory (CADRI, Wolfe et al., 2001; 35 two-part items). Of these three, the Safe Dates Scale and CADRI were developed specifically for adolescents. The CTS-2 and CADRI assess sexual violence, in addition to psychological and physical violence. All three scales assess victimization and perpetration. The CADRI uses gender specific language and thus measures violence in heterosexual relationships; therefore, the CADRI commonly is adapted to include gender-neutral language (Smith et al., in press).

The most widely used measure of sexual violence is the Sexual Experiences Survey (SES, Koss & Gidycz, 1985; 10 items). This measure captures sexual violence by any perpetrator, including dating partners, and is available in two versions, one for perpetration and one for victimization.

It should be noted that the measures described above are typically used in research and evaluation, whereas in clinical settings either victim disclosures or health-provider administered assessment instruments are primarily used to detect violence.

Programs That Prevent Dating and Sexual Violence Among Youth

A recent upsurge in programs with evidence of effectiveness in preventing some form of dating or sexual violence among adolescents addresses long-standing gaps in the field, namely that programs traditionally have targeted and changed attitudes (Ting, 2009) and that very few programs achieve reductions in dating and sexual violence perpetration (Whitaker et al., 2006). Although more work is needed, the increase in rigorous evaluations conducted in the past decade (for reviews, see De Koker, Matthews, Zuch, Bastien, & Mason-Jones, 2014; DeGue et al., 2014) gives practitioners a menu of programs from which to choose. Moreover, many of the programs are tailored for specific groups of at-risk youth, such as athletes (e.g., *Coaching Boys into Men)* or youth who have experienced child maltreatment (e.g., *Youth Relationships Project)*, which may serve to meet the unique needs of particular schools or communities.

The ten programs that have evidence of effectiveness in individual studies for preventing verbal, physical, and/or sexual dating violence among adolescents using a randomized controlled trial or quasi-experimental design are described in Table 13.2. Six of the programs are implemented during the school day (*SD, SB, 4th R, RS+, IYG*) or after school (*CBIM)* by school staff. Three programs are implemented in the community (*BALL, YRP*, and *SS)*. One program (*FSD*) is implemented by mail, such that participating families receive booklets in the mail, which include dating violence prevention information and activities that parents/caregivers and youth complete together. This novel approach enables parents/caregivers to complete the prevention activities at their convenience and overcomes a primary complication of family-focused programs—parent engagement and availability. All of the programs except for *SB* use a curricula or multi-session format. The effective component of *SB* employs a three-pronged school-level intervention that raises awareness of dating violence through posters, assists school personnel in monitoring areas in the school where youth feel unsafe ("hot spot" mapping), and equips school personnel to maintain separation among youth in unhealthy and/or unsafe relationships though "respecting boundary agreements," which are school-based versions of restraining orders.

Only two programs (*SD* and *SB*) have clear evidence of preventing sexual violence perpetration by a dating partner (*SD*) or peer (*SB*). *CBIM* and *SS* both used a composite measure of dating violence that included sexual violence, but because the items were combined with other forms of dating violence, it is not possible to know if reductions in violence were found for sexual violence specifically. In addition, as noted in Table 13.2, some programs have effects on other risk behaviors, such as weapon carrying and peer violence.

A major limitation of these programs is that all ten programs have only been evaluated in one trial, typically by the program developer. Replication of effects by independent evaluators is needed. In addition, a recent review and meta-analysis suggest the clinical significance of these interventions may be small (De La Rue, Polanin, Espelage, & Piggot, 2014; Fellmeth et al., 2013) and therefore, results of single studies should be interpreted with caution. Many other dating and sexual violence prevention programs exist, but either they have not been evaluated, have been evaluated and show no behavior change, or have been evaluated and show

TABLE 13.2 Overview of Programs with Evidence of Preventing Dating and/or Sexual Violence Victimization or Perpetration among Youth

Program	*Evaluation(s)*	*Program Description*	*Sample*	*Design*	*Setting*	*Forms of dating violence assessed*	*Behavioral Effects*	*Additional Information*
Youth-Focused								
Safe Dates (SD)	Foshee et al., 1998, 2004	10 sessions in addition to play and poster contest. Program content addresses gender stereotyping, conflict management skills, dating violence norms, and belief in the need for help and awareness of services.	8th and 9th grade youth from rural North Carolina	RCT	School	Psychological, physical, and sexual dating violence victimization and perpetration	Prevented psychological, physical, and sexual violence perpetration in current relationship at 1-month follow-up; Effects varied based on youth's previous experiences with violence; At 4-year follow-up program participants reported less physical and sexual violence perpetration and victimization than non-participants.	Effects mediated by norms, gender stereotyping, constructive communication, constructive anger response, and awareness of services; Positive effects have also been found for peer violence and weapon carrying (Foshee et al., 2014). All youth in the trial were exposed to community activities that involved training providers and offering services for youth in violent relationships.

4th R: Skills for Youth Relationships (4th R)	Wolfe et al., 2009	21 sessions Program content included personal safety and injury prevention, healthy growth and sexuality, and substance use prevention.	9th grade youth from rural and urban Canada	RCT	School	Physical dating violence perpetration	Prevented physical dating violence perpetration for boys (not girls) at 2.5-year follow-up; increased boys' condom use.	Intended to be a school's health curriculum, often tailored by developers to meet specific academic requirements; cost estimated to be $16/student. Program not effective for preventing peer violence or substance use.
Shifting Boundaries (SB)	Taylor, Stein, Mumford, & Woods, 2013	6-session curricula and school-level intervention Classroom curricula included content on legal consequences of perpetration, healthy relationships, and gender roles. School-level intervention included: posters, hot-spot mapping, and building-based restraining orders.	Middle school youth from New York City	RCT	School	Sexual harassment perpetration and victimization; Sexual and physical violence victimization and perpetration (involving peers or dating partners)	School-level intervention prevented sexual harassment, victimization, and perpetration; peer sexual violence perpetration and victimization; and sexual dating violence victimization at 6-month follow-up.	No significant effects for classroom curricula.

(Continued)

TABLE 13.2 (Continued)

Program	*Evaluation(s)*	*Program Description*	*Sample*	*Design*	*Setting*	*Forms of dating violence assessed*	*Behavioral Effects*	*Additional Information*
It's Your Game . . . Keep It Real	Peskin et al., 2014	24-session classroom and computer-based program (12 sessions in 7th grade, 12 in 8th grade) that aims to delay sexual behavior and promote healthy dating behaviors. Program also includes 6 parent-child homework activities.	7th and 8th grade youth from urban schools	RCT	School	Physical and emotional dating violence victimization and perpetration	Prevented physical dating violence victimization and emotional dating violence, victimization among boys, and girls and emotional dating violence perpetration among boys.	Effects on dating violence varied by race/ethnicity. Program also showed effects delaying initiation of sex and reduced other sexual risk behaviors.
Coaching Boys into Men (CBIM)	Miller et al., 2012, 2013	11 "training cards" used by coaches to lead 10–15 minute discussions with male athletes during practice.	Male high school athletes from urban schools	RCT	During after school sports practice	Composite measure, including male-to-female emotional, physical, and	Prevented dating violence perpetration at 1-year follow-up (not at 3-month).	

		Program content targets gender and dating violence norms and bystander behaviors.				sexual dating violence perpetration		
Stepping Stones (SS)	Jewkes et al., 2008	50-hour program administered over 6–8 weeks. Program content included a variety of sexual health topics, gender-based violence, grief and loss, and communication skills.	15–26-year-olds in rural South Africa	RCT	Community	Composite measure, including physical or sexual partner violence perpetration	Prevented partner violence perpetration among men at 24-month follow-up (not at 12-month follow-up); Also prevented new herpes infections, transactional sex, and problem drinking among male participants.	Unclear if women were assessed for violence victimization or perpetration, although no effects for women's violence were found. Female program participants engaged in more transactional sex than non-participants at 12-month follow-up.
Youth Relationships Project (YRP)	Wolfe et al. 2003	18 sessions delivered by community professionals (e.g., social worker).	14–16-year-olds at-risk youth with histories of child mal-treatment	RCT	Community	Perpetration and victimization of physical and emotional violence and	Prevented physical violence perpetration and emotional and physical violence victimization,	Non-program participants evidenced decreases in victimization and perpetration as well, but program

(*Continued*)

TABLE 13.2 (Continued)

Program	*Evaluation(s)*	*Program Description*	*Sample*	*Design*	*Setting*	*Forms of dating violence assessed*	*Behavioral Effects*	*Additional Information*
		Program content includes awareness of abuse, interpersonal problem solving and communication skills, and gender-role expectations.				threatening behaviors	as well as threatening behavior victimization, at 2-year follow-up.	participants evidence a steeper decline on specified outcomes.
Building a Lasting Love (BALL)	Langhinrichsen-Rohling & Turner, 2012	4 sessions Program content included emotion regulation, stress management, and communication skills, as well as knowledge of relationship violence and safety planning.	High-risk urban African American girls receiving pregnancy services	Quasi-experimental	Community (family planning clinic)	Psychological, mild and severe physical violence perpetration and victimization	Prevented psychological violence perpetration and severe physical violence victimization.	Small sample size.
Relationship Smarts Plus (RS+)	Adler-Baeder, Kerpelman, Schramm, Higginbotham, & Paulk, 2007	12 sessions Program content includes knowledge and skills related to healthy and unhealthy dating.	High school youth across Alabama	Quasi-experimental	School	Verbal and physical dating violence	Prevented verbal aggression perpetration at post-test (2 months following pre-test).	

Family-Focused								
Families for Safe Dates (FSD)	Foshee et al., 2012	6 booklets (introduction booklet for parents/caregivers + 5 booklets to complete with youth) mailed to participating families once every two weeks Booklets contain information and activities related to dating violence knowledge and attitudes, youth conflict resolution skills, and parent/caregiver monitoring and date rule setting for youth.	National sample	RCT	Mail with health educator phone follow-up	Physical dating violence victimization and perpetration	Prevented physical dating violence victimization among youth whose parents participated in program at 3-month follow-up.	Offshoots of this program are currently being evaluated for 1) mothers who have experienced domestic violence and their children, and 2) for Latino families.

Note. RCT = Randomized Controlled Trial.

harmful effects (DeGue et al., 2014; Whitaker et al., 2006). Therefore, programs with evidence of effectiveness should be used first. If intended effects are not obtained, then evidence-informed programs—or programs that reflect the principles of prevention (e.g., use varied teaching methods, are theory driven, employ well-trained staff; Nation et al., 2003) and known risk and protective factors (Teten Tharp, DeGue et al., 2013; Vagi et al., 2013) but have yet to be evaluated—may be considered. The recent increase in programs with evidence of preventing violence is promising and foreshadows a new era in dating and sexual violence prevention in which schools and communities have multiple options for successfully preventing violence and promoting healthy relationships among youth.

Emerging Approaches to Prevention

Another limitation of the programs in Table 13.2 is that each program only targets one level of the social ecology (individual, family, school/community, or society). Although *SB* includes both a classroom and school-level component, only the school-level component contributed to youth behavior change. Although *SD* included community activities in the trial, both conditions received these activities, so it is unclear if they contributed to the effectiveness of the program. In addition, although *FSD* is sold by the publisher with *SD*, the two programs are often not implemented together. Therefore, a gap exists for programs that address the broader social-ecological contexts in which youth are embedded. As outlined in Table 13.1, because youth may experience risk for dating or sexual violence in multiple contexts, such as with friends, at school, or in their family, prevention is needed that takes these different contexts into account. Recent work is addressing this gap, by building comprehensive, multi-level prevention around evidence-based programs. These comprehensive approaches use a healthy relationship framework (Teten Tharp, Carter et al., 2013) and engage youth, their peers, parents, teachers, and community. A hallmark of these programs is that they initiate prevention in middle school, in order to stop violence before it begins. Two examples exist: Robert Wood Johnson Foundation's *Start Strong: Building Healthy Teen Relationships* and the Centers for Disease Control and Prevention's *Dating Matters®: Strategies to Promote Healthy Teen Relationships*.

Start Strong was implemented in 2008–2012 in 11 sites across the United States through a variety of community-based and public agencies. Communities used *SD* or *4th R* as the school curricula and developed additional strategies to engage youth and their parents, as well as working for policy-level changes to support dating violence prevention in schools. The evaluation of *Start Strong* suggests the combination of prevention approaches had short-term (fall to spring of grade 7) positive effects on parent-child communication and youth dating relationship satisfaction and support; short and long-term (fall of grade 7 to spring of grade 8) decreases in gender stereotypes and attitudes supporting dating violence were also found (Miller et al., 2014).

Dating Matters® (Teten Tharp et al., 2011) is a comprehensive approach for dating violence prevention that was designed for youth in high risk urban communities. The *Dating Matters®* approach is built on *SD and FSD* and provides prevention strategies for youth, their parents, and educators throughout middle school, in addition to equipping local health departments to inform local policy for dating violence prevention and engaging youth via social media. From 2011–2016, *Dating Matters®* is being implemented and evaluated for effects on dating and sexual violence perpetration and victimization in four urban communities across the United States in a randomized controlled trial. Data from the *Dating Matters®* baseline survey underscore the need for prevention among youth in high risk urban communities; among middle school youth who had ever dated, 32% reported perpetrating physical violence, 20% reported threatening a partner, and 15% reported perpetrating sexual violence at some time in their lives (Niolon et al., 2015). Starting in 2014, *Dating Matters®* tools and strategies will be made available to other schools or communities interested in implementing comprehensive programs that promote healthy relationships (see below for resources from *Dating Matters®* and *Start Strong*).

Summary and Conclusions

Dating and sexual violence affect far too many middle and high school youth and are associated with a variety of negative consequences, including poor academic performance and re-victimization in college. An opportunity exists to implement effective prevention programs in middle and high school. Effective prevention takes into account the risk and protective factors of the target audience and uses strategies that have been proven to reduce violent behavior in rigorous evaluations. Emerging, comprehensive approaches engage youth, parents, educators, schools, and communities, and demonstrate that everyone has a role in preventing dating and sexual violence. Using this best available research, youth, their families, schools, and communities can work together to foster and support healthy and safe youth relationships.

Take-Home Points

- Dating and sexual violence among school-aged youth are serious problems that are associated with poor academic performance and other negative consequences.
- Schools can have multiple positive influences on dating and sexual violence:
    - Educators can identify the risk factors and warning signs of violence.
    - Educators can know resources to help survivors.
    - Attachment to and engagement in school protects young people from becoming perpetrators of violence.
    - Violence is preventable and schools can use a variety of effective approaches to keep youth safe and healthy.

- Emerging approaches, such as Start Strong and Dating Matters, combine school-based strategies with family-based, community-based, and policy-oriented prevention.

Resources

- National Teen Dating Abuse Helpline: www.loveisrespect.org
  - Call: 1–866–331–9474, Text: "loveis" to 22522, TTY: 1–866–331–8453,
- National Sexual Assault Telephone and Online Hotlines: http://apps.rainn.org/ohl-bridge/
  - Call 1–800–656-HOPE (4673)
- Centers for Disease Control and Prevention Veto Violence Online Trainings (e.g., *Dating Matters: Understanding Teen Dating Violence*, *Principles of Prevention*): www.vetoviolence.org
- Lessons Learned from Start Strong: http://startstrong.futureswithoutviolence.org/
- The School Health Index: http://www.cdc.gov/HealthyYouth/SHI/
- Assessing victimization: http://www.cdc.gov/violenceprevention/pdf/ipv/ipvandsvscreening.pdf

References

Adler-Baeder, F., Kerpelman, J.L., Schramm, D.G., Higginbotham, B., & Paulk, A. (2007). The impact of relationship education on adolescents of diverse backgrounds. *Family Relations*, *56*, 291–303.

Archer, J. (2002). Sex differences in physically aggressive acts between heterosexual partners: A meta-analytic review. *Aggression and Violent Behavior*, 7, 313–351.

Banyard, V.L., & Cross, C. (2008). Consequences of teen dating violence: Understanding intervening variables in ecological context. *Violence Against Women*, *14*, 998–1013.

Basile, K.C., Black, M.C., Simon, T.R., Arias, I., Brener, N.D., & Saltzman, L.E. (2006). The association between self-reported lifetime history of forced sexual intercourse and recent health-risk behaviors: Findings from the 2003 National Youth Risk Behavior Survey. *Journal of Adolescent Health*, 39, 752.e1–752.e7 (available online only).

Basile, K.C., Smith, S.G., Breiding, M.J., Black, M.C., & Mahendra, R.R. (2015). *Sexual violence surveillance: Uniform definitions and recommended data elements, Version 2.0.* Atlanta, GA: National Center for Injury Prevention and Control, Centers for Disease Control and Prevention.

Black, M.C., Basile, K.C., Breiding, M.J., Smith, S.G., Walters, M.L., Merrick, M.T., . . . Stevens, M.R. (2011). *The national intimate partner and sexual violence survey (NISVS): 2010 summary report.* Atlanta, GA: National Center for Injury Prevention and Control, Centers for Disease Control and Prevention.

Borowsky, L.M., Hogan, M., & Ireland, M. (1997). Adolescent sexual aggression: Risk and protective factors. *Pediatrics*, *100*, 1–8.

Breiding, M.J., Chen J., & Black, M.C. (2014). *Intimate partner violence in the United States—2010.* Atlanta, GA: National Center for Injury Prevention and Control, Centers for Disease Control and Prevention.

Centers for Disease Control and Prevention (CDC). (2014). *Understanding teen dating violence: Fact sheet.* Atlanta, GA: National Center for Injury Prevention and Control, Centers for Disease Control and Prevention.

Cleveland, H.H., Herrera, V.M., & Stuewig, J. (2003). Abusive males and abused females in adolescent relationships: Risk factor similarity and dissimilarity and the role of relationship seriousness. *Journal of Family Violence, 18*, 325–339.

De La Rue, L., Polanin, J.R., Espelage, D.L., & Piggot, T.D. (2014). School-based interventions to reduce dating and sexual violence: A systematic review. *Campbell Systematic Reviews,* 7. doi: 10.4073/csr.2014.7

DeGue, S., Valle, L.A., Holt, M., Massetti, G., Matjasko, J., & Teten Tharp, A. (2014). A systematic review of primary prevention strategies for sexual violence perpetration. *Aggression and Violent Behavior, 19*, 346–362.

De Koker, P., Matthews, C., Zuch, M., Bastien, S., & Mason-Jones, A.K. (2014). A systematic review of interventions for preventing adolescent intimate partner violence. *Journal of Adolescent Health, 54*, 3–13.

Fellmeth, G.L.T., Heffernan, C., Nurse, J., Habibula, S., & Sethi, D. (2013). Educational and skills-based interventions for preventing relationship and dating violence in adolescents and young adults. *Cochrane Database of Systematic Reviews 2013*, Issue 6. Art. No.: CD004534. doi: 10.1002/14651858.CD004534.pub3

Foshee, V.A., Bauman, K.E., Arriaga, X.B., Helms, R.W., Koch, G.G., Linger, G.F. (1998). An evaluation of safe dates, an adolescent dating violence prevention program. *American Journal of Public Health, 88*, 45–50.

Foshee, V.A., Bauman, K.E., Ennett S.T., Linder, F., Benefield, T., & Suchindran, C. (2004). Assessing the long-term effects of the Safe Dates Program and a Booster in preventing and reducing adolescent dating violence victimization and perpetration. *American Journal of Public Health, 94*, 619–624.

Foshee, V.A., Linder, G., Bauman, K.E., Langwick, S.A., Arriaga, X.B., Heath, J.L., & Bangdiwala, S. (1996). The Safe Dates Project: Theoretical basis, evaluation design, and selected baseline findings. *American Journal of Preventive Medicine, 12*, 39–47.

Foshee, V.A., McNaughton Reyes, L., Agnew-Brune, C.B., Simon, T.R., Vagi, K., Lee, R., & Suchindran, C. (2014). The effects of the evidence-based Safe Dates dating abuse prevention program on other youth violence outcomes. *Prevention Science, 15*, 907–916.

Foshee, V.A., Reyes, H.L.M., Ennett, S.T., Cance, J.D., Bauman, K.E., & Bowling, J.M. (2012). Assessing the effects of Families for Safe Dates, a family-based teen dating abuse prevention program. *Journal of Adolescent Health, 51*, 349–356.

Holmes, M.M., Resnick, H.S., Kilpatrick, D.G., & Best, C.L. (1996). Rape-related pregnancy: estimates and descriptive characteristics from a national sample of women. *American Journal of Obstetrics and Gynecology, 175*, 320–324.

Jewkes, R., Nduna, M., Levin, J., Jama, N., Dunkle, K., Puren, A. & Duvvury, N. (2008). Impact of Stepping Stones on incidence of HIV and HSV-2 and sexual behavior in rural South Africa: Cluster randomized controlled trial. *British Medical Journal, 337*, a506.

Jewkes, R., Sen, P., & Garcia-Moreno, C. (2002). Sexual violence. In E. Krug, L.L. Dahlberg, J.A. Mercy et al. (Eds.), *World report on violence and health* (pp. 213–239). Geneva, Switzerland: World Health Organization.

Kann, L., Kinchen, S., Shanklin, S.L., Flint, K.H., Kawkins, J., Harris, W.A., . . . Centers for Disease Control and Prevention (CDC). (2014). Youth risk behavior surveillance—United States 2013. *MMWR, 63(No. SS-#4)*, 1–169.

Koss, M.P., & Gidycz, C.A. (1985). Sexual Experiences Survey: Reliability and validity. *Journal of Consulting and Clinical Psychology, 53*, 422–423.

Langhinrichsen-Rohling, J., & Turner, L.A. (2012). The efficacy of an intimate partner violence prevention program with high-risk adolescent girls: A preliminary test. *Prevention Science, 13*, 384–394.

Luo, F., Stone, D., & Teten Tharp, A. (2014). Physical dating violence victimization among sexual minority youth. *American Journal of Public Health, 104*, e66–e73.

Miller, E., Tancredi, D.J., McCauley, H.L., Decker, M.R., Catrina, M., Anderson, H.A., . . . Silverman, J. (2013). One year follow-up pf a coach-delivered dating violence prevention program: A cluster randomized controlled trial. *American Journal of Preventive Medicine, 45*, 108–112.

Miller, E., Tancredi, D.J., McCauley, H.L., Decker, M.R., Virata, M.C.D., Anderson, H.A., . . . Silverman, J.G. (2012). "Coaching boys into men": A cluster-randomized controlled trial of a dating violence prevention program. *Journal of Adolescent Health, 51*, 431–438.

Miller, S., Williams, J., Cutbush, S., Gibbs, D., Clinton-Sherrod, M., & Jones, S. (2014). Evaluation of the *Start Strong* Initiative: Preventing teen dating violence and promoting healthy relationships among middle school students. Unpublished manuscript/under review.

Nation, M., Crusto, C., Wandersman, A., Kumpfer, K.L., Seybolt, D., Morrissey-Kane, E., & Davino, K. (2003). What works in prevention: Principles of effective prevention programs. *American Psychologist, 58*, 449–456.

Niolon, P.H., Tharp, A.T., Latzman, N.E., Vivolo-Kantor, A., Valle, L.A., Burton, T., . . . Kuoh, H. (2015). The "Dating Matters®: Strategies to Promote Healthy Teen Relationships" approach: Using a comprehensive strategy to target teen dating violence and a constellation of risk factors among youth, *Journal of Adolescent Health, 56*, s5–13.

O'Leary, K.D., & Slep, A.M.S. (2012). Prevention of partner violence by focusing on behaviors of both young males and females. *Prevention Science, 13*, 329–339.

Peskin, M.F., Markham, C.M., Shegog, R., Baumier, E.R., Addy, R.C., Tortolero, S.R. (2014). Effects of the It's Your Game . . . Keep It Real program on dating violence in ethnic-minority middle school youths: A group randomized trial. *American Journal of Public Health, 104*, 1471–1477.

Smith, J., Mulford, C., Latzman, N., Teten Tharp, A., Niolon, P., & Blachman-Demner, D. (in press). Taking stock of behavioral measures of adolescent dating violence. *Journal of Aggression, Maltreatment and Trauma.*

Straus, M.A., Hamby, S.L., Boney-McCoy, S., & Sugarman, D.B. (1996). The revised conflict tactics scale (CTS2). *Journal of Family Issues, 17*, 283–316.

Taylor, B.G., Stein, N.D., Mumford, E.A., & Woods, D. (2013). Shifting boundaries: An experimental evaluation of a dating violence prevention program in middle schools. *Prevention Science, 14*, 64–76.

Teten, A.L., Ball, B, Valle, L.A., Noonan, R., & Rosenbluth, B. (2009). Considerations for the definition, measurement, consequences, and prevention of dating violence victimization among adolescent girls. *Journal of Women's Health, 18*, 923–927.

Teten Tharp, A., Burton, T., Freire, K., Hall, D., Harrier, S., Latzman, N., . . . Vagi, K. (2011). Dating Matters™: Strategies to Promote Healthy Teen Relationships. *Journal of Women's Health, 20*, 1–5.

Teten Tharp, A., Carter, M., Fasula, A., Hatfield-Timajchy, K., Jayne, P., Latzman, N., & Kinsey, J. (2013). Advancing sexual and reproductive health by promoting healthy relationships. *Journal of Women's Health, 22*, 1–4.

Teten Tharp, A., DeGue, S., Valle, L.A., Matjasko, J., Massetti, G.M., & Brookmeyer, K. (2013). A qualitative systematic review of risk and protective factors for sexual violence perpetration. *Trauma, Violence, and Abuse, 14*, 133–167.

Ting, S.R. (2009). Meta-analysis on dating violence prevention among middle and high schools. *Journal of School Violence, 8*, 328–337.

Vagi, K.J., Rothman, E., Latzman, N.E., Teten Tharp, A., Hall, D.M., & Breiding, M. (2013). Beyond correlates: A review of risk and protective factors for adolescent dating violence perpetration. *Journal of Youth and Adolescence, 42*, 633–649.

Whitaker, D.J., Morrison, S., Lindquist, C., Hawkins, S.R., O'Neil, J.A., & Nesius, A.M. (2006). A critical review of interventions for the primary prevention of perpetration of dating violence. *Aggression and Violent Behavior, 11*, 151–166.

Wolfe, D.A., Crooks, C., Jaffe, P., Chiodo, D., Hughes, R., Ellis, W., . . . Donner, A. (2009). A school-based program to prevent adolescent dating violence: A cluster randomized trial. *Archives of Pediatrics and Adolescent Medicine, 163*, 692–699.

Wolfe, D.A., Scott, K., Reitzel-Jaffe, D., Wekerle, C., Grasley, C., & Straatman, A.L. (2001). Development and validation of the conflict in adolescent dating relationships inventory. *Psychological Assessment, 13*, 277–293.

Wolfe, D.A., Wekerle, C., Scott, K., Straatman, A., Grasley, C., & Reitzel-Jaffe, D. (2003). Dating violence prevention with at-risk youth: A controlled outcome evaluation. *Journal of Consulting & Clinical Psychology, 71*, 279–291.

14

EFFECTS OF CHILDHOOD TRAUMATIC EVENT EXPERIENCES

Joseph R. Cohen and Carla Kmett Danielson

Dating back to the early 1980s, systematic investigations into the prevalence and consequences of experiencing trauma have shed light onto how millions of youth are impacted by these events (Costello, Erkanli, Fairbank, & Angold, 2002). The term "trauma" refers to a myriad of negative contexts that may be experienced during childhood and adolescence, including domestic violence, medical trauma, natural disasters, community violence, school violence, neglect, physical abuse, refugee and war zone trauma, sexual abuse, terrorism, and traumatic grief. Although rates of most childhood traumatic events (CTEs) in the United States are declining (Finkelhor, Turner, Hamby, & Ormrod, 2014), CTEs are still a part of life for the majority of American youth (Saunders & Adams, 2014). Thus, greater awareness of CTE and its effects in school settings is essential (Slade & Wissow, 2007).

Academic Consequences of Maltreatment

Maltreatment represents the most studied form of trauma experienced by youth. Although definitions for maltreatment vary across legal, professional, and cultural contexts, there is general consensus around four domains: (1) *Physical Abuse*: Non-accidental infliction of injury on the child; (2) *Sexual Abuse*: Attempted or actual sexual contact with a child for a person's sexual satisfaction or financial benefit; (3) *Neglect*: Failure to provide for the child's basic needs; and (4) *Emotional maltreatment*: Extreme thwarting of children's basic emotional needs (Cicchetti & Banny, 2014). These definitions, together with rigorous, prospective study designs, have led to a better understanding of the direct and indirect impact of maltreatment.

School providers may witness the deleterious consequences of maltreatment starting at a young age. Miller, Flynn, and Vandermeulen (2008) found that by age

4, maltreated children were 6 times more likely to be receiving special education services compared to children in the general population. In kindergarten, children with maltreatment histories begin to show lower cognitive, reading, and mathematics scores (Crozier & Barth, 2005). Although academic outcome differences are greatest for children in lower grades (Flynn, Ghazal, Legault, Vandermeulen, & Petrick, 2004; Leiter, 2007), systematic differences between maltreated and non-maltreated youth persist into late childhood/adolescence. Kurtz, Gaudin, Wodarski, and Howing (1993) found that maltreated children and adolescents had more school absences and poorer school performance, and over half of the physically abused (55%) and neglected (60%) youth needed to repeat a grade.

Recent research suggests that neglected youth may be at particular risk for cognitive deficits and academic failure (Romano, Babchishin, Marquis, & Fréchette, 2014). Neglected youth struggle academically throughout childhood and adolescence as evidenced by lower grades, higher teacher ratings of learning problems, higher grade repeats, and more school absences compared to both non-maltreated youth and physically and sexually abused youth (Fantuzzo, Perlman, & Dobbins, 2011; Kazemian, Widom, & Farrington, 2011). Language development may underlie these academic difficulties, as neglected infants and preschoolers demonstrate problems in expressive and receptive language (Moreno-Manso, García-Baamonde, Alonso, & Barona, 2010). It is posited that *emotional neglect* (the failure of a parent to attend to a child's basic emotional needs) may be particularly damaging as inconsistent responses from a caregiver leads to confusion in youth and consequently an avoidance of expressing oneself (Katz, 1992; Moreno-Manso et al., 2010). Within the classroom setting, this may manifest in increased academic difficulties, as well as the inability to express the need for help.

Mental Health Consequences of Maltreatment

Along with school impairment, psychological distress is also an associated consequence of maltreatment experiences. Consistent with the principles of *multifinality* (i.e., multiple possible outcomes from a single event/vulnerability; Cicchetti & Rogosch, 1996), maltreatment is linked with a broad set of psychological symptoms. Slade and Wissow (2007) posit a model that: (1) links childhood maltreatment to academic difficulties and poor mental health, (2) a bidirectional relation in which academic difficulties mediate the relation between childhood maltreatment and poor mental health, and likewise, mental health issues explain the relation between maltreatment and academic performance. Thus, an understanding of common CTE-related mental health symptoms can help school providers contextualize students' behavior.

Internalizing disorders are a common psychological sequelae for maltreated youth. Recent meta-analyses show that maltreatment predicts a severe course of treatment-resistant depression (Nanni, Uher, & Danese, 2012). Decreases in self-esteem and self-agency may explain the relation between maltreatment experiences and depression (Kim & Cicchetti, 2006). Anxiety disorders (Stein, Schork, & Gelernter, 2007) and posttraumatic stress disorder (PTSD; Cloitre et al., 2009), are also commonly associated with childhood maltreatment. With regard to PTSD, evidence suggests that maltreated youth suffering from these symptoms are at heightened risk for suicide compared to maltreated youth not experiencing PTSD (Lopez-Castroman et al., 2014). Incident characteristics, such as age of onset, duration/severity of maltreatment, and multiple forms of maltreatment (i.e., polyvictimization), increase one's odds of developing emotional distress (Manly, Kim, Rogosch, & Cicchetti, 2001).

In addition to internalizing disorders, it is common for a wide range of behavioral disorders to present in adolescence among maltreated youth. In a multi-wave, longitudinal study, Egeland, Yates, Appleyard, and van Dulmen (2002) demonstrated how physical abuse in early childhood led to alienation in preschool, which then predicted externalizing problems in elementary school, and eventual antisocial behavior in adolescence. These types of models, which examine the sequential consequences of negative events across development, are commonly referred to as *developmental cascades* (Masten & Cicchetti, 2010) and demonstrate the link between early childhood adversity and prospective, heterogeneous outcomes.

Developmental cascade models help explain why certain youth may go on to develop externalizing symptoms later in life, as opposed to emotional distress. Attachment relationships, development of the self-system, and peer relations (Cicchetti & Banny, 2014) are just some of the developmental consequences from child maltreatment that can dictate psychological outcomes later in life. The development of aggression represents a core aspect of several cascade models in maltreated youth. Aggressive responses stemming from social cognitive deficits (see Tiesl & Cicchetti, 2008) seem to contribute to limited friend networks (Howe & Parke, 2001) and frequent bullying paradigms (both as perpetrator and victim; Shields & Cicchetti, 2001). Specifically, maltreated boys may respond with more *physically* aggressive acts to teachers and peers, while maltreated girls may tend to respond with more *relational* aggression (Cullerton-Sen et al., 2008). Intervening with these aggressive behaviors may represent a critical step towards distinguishing between long-term maladaptive and resilient responses following a CTE.

CTEs in Urban School Settings

Although CTEs are common across youth populations (Finkelhor, Turner, Shattuck, & Hamby, 2013), youth living in urban settings are at particular risk. According to the United States Department of Justice, up to 98% of youth living in an urban environment are exposed to some form of violent crime (Snyder & Sickmund, 2006). Community violence, which includes direct victimization (e.g., threatened, beaten up, shot, assaulted), witnessing any of these acts, or hearing/learning about these violent crimes (e.g., vicarious exposure; Buka et al.,

2001), is something most American children and adolescents living in an urban environment will experience (Overstreet & Mathews, 2011). PTSD is the most common clinical outcome in community violence-exposed youth (Fowler et al., 2009). Research suggests that living in a neighborhood in which youth fear for their own and family's safety (Overstreet & Mathews, 2011), leaves children and adolescents chronically "on guard" and hyperaroused, leading to the emergence of PTSD symptoms (Schell, Marshall, & Jaycox, 2004).

Externalizing symptoms are also associated with community violence, especially for those who were either the victim or directly witnessed the event (Fowler et al., 2009). Youth exposed to community violence tend to engage in greater bullying perpetration in school compared to their peers (Low & Espelage, 2014). Social cognition theory suggests that this may happen because youth directly exposed to community violence interpret aggressive behavior as a problem-solving method, and begin to adapt some of these strategies themselves (Guerra et al., 2003). With regard to depression and anxiety and a connection with community violence, the findings are less clear. Some research posits that chronic violence exposure can lead to posttraumatic symptoms that lead to other emotional and behavioral problems (Kolk, 2005; Overstreet & Mathews, 2011); however, other findings suggest that youth become emotionally desensitized to chronic violence and other health indices are needed to better capture the negative impact of community violence (Rosenfield, Jouriles, McDonald, & Mueller, 2014).

Community violence exposure also relates to poorer academic outcomes (e.g., GPA; Voisin, Neilands, & Hunnicut, 2011) and reduced school engagement (e.g., school enjoyment; Janosz et al., 2008). Symptoms of psychological distress may help explain this relation. For instance, youth with PTSD may experience intrusive thoughts related to the violent event that prevents them from concentrating in school. Children who observed community violence in their classroom may also refuse to attend school to avoid reminders of the traumatic event (Mathews, Dempsey, & Overstreet, 2009). In addition to psychological distress, impaired neurobiological development in domains related to sustained attention, memory, and executive functioning in youth chronically exposed to community violence may explain poor academic outcomes (Overstreet & Mathews, 2011).

Traumatic grief is a related form of CTE that urban school providers may be likely to encounter. Although an emerging area of research, initial findings suggest that traumatic grief represents a serious public health threat for pediatric emotional distress (Kaplow, Howell, & Layne, 2014). Similar to other forms of CTE, the psychological and academic impact of traumatic grief depends on pre-existing familial and individual factors, and circumstances surrounding the death (Kaplow et al., 2014). However, as research continues to amass in this area, specific treatment protocols are being augmented to target symptoms of depression and PTSD in youth who have not only experienced a CTE, but are also coping with the loss of a loved one (Cohen, Mannarino, & Deblinger, 2012).

Special Issues in Trauma

School violence, defined as examples of community violence experienced within school, is an area of growing interest within the trauma field. Although bullying is one form of school violence, the most tragic examples are school suicides and school shootings (i.e., lethal school violence; LSV). With regard to LSV, the psychological toll on students can be immense. Many students exposed to LSV develop psychological distress and academic impairment characteristic of responses to other CTEs. Past research demonstrated that from childhood through late adolescence (i.e., university-aged students), LSV results in poorer academic performance and school attendance (Daniels & Bradley, 2011). In response, protocols have been developed to help students, and schools as a whole, cope in the aftermath of LSV (Jaycox, Stein, & Wong, 2014).

Although a smaller body of literature, findings are also startling concerning school suicides. Opposed to other cohorts, adolescents may be especially susceptible to "suicide clusters," where one suicide leads to a series of suicides in the community (Haw, Hawton, Niedzwiedz, & Platt, 2013). Suicides within the school, where the impact can be more direct, may be even more deleterious to adolescents' mental health (Kaplow et al., 2014). Therefore, school personnel need to be proactive with adolescents who may have lost a peer/loved one due to suicide. Similar to LSV, several school-based protocols have been developed for how to best prevent, treat, and respond to suicidal ideation within the school context (Robinson et al., 2013).

Finally, understanding mental health outcomes in adolescents following natural disasters has become a growing area of interest within the CTE literature (Furr, Comer, Edmunds, & Kendall, 2010). School-based interventions have been developed to help students cope with trauma-related stress following a natural disaster (e.g., Weems et al., 2009). Social support seems to be a key predictor of post-disaster functioning (Furr et al., 2010). As natural disasters may impact traditional systems of support for youth, school providers can play an increased role for children following a natural disaster.

Assessing for Trauma and Trauma Effects

Assessment is a critical step towards providing competent trauma-related services within any practice setting. Elements of a competent trauma assessment incorporate many of the central elements for any mental health assessment with youth: fostering a therapeutic alliance; use of objective and psychometrically sound measures; behavioral observations; and collateral information from caregivers, teachers, and any other significant adults in the child's life (Kisiel, Conradi, Fehrenbach, Torgerson, & Briggs, 2014). However, there are additional considerations that are unique to trauma assessments and deserve consideration within this context.

Assessing for a range of traumatic events is critical for any comprehensive trauma assessment. Because past trauma experiences influence the impact of future trauma experiences (Margolin & Vickerman, 2007), and polyvictimization is the norm rather than the exception (Finkelhor, Ormrod, & Turner, 2007), having a chronological understanding of any acute or chronic traumas in the past is vital. Inherent in assessing the nature of current and past traumas is gaining a firm understanding of the possible family impact/dynamics in light of the trauma (Kisiel et al., 2014). Understanding the various ecological systems impacted by the trauma can provide insight into subsequent stressors the student may be coping with since the traumatic event. Finally, it is critical to use behavior-specific terminology when assessing for traumatic events. Past research shows significant underreporting of traumatic events when using latent terminology (e.g., the word "rape") as opposed to behavioral specific words (e.g., "penetration") during the assessment process (Resnick, Kilpatrick, Dansky, Saunders, & Best, 1993).

One of the more difficult aspects of completing a trauma assessment is balancing questions about traumatic events and inquiries into the patient's mental health. The need for intricate knowledge for both of these domains is why most trauma assessments take 2–3 sessions (Kisiel et al., 2014). As reviewed above, trauma assessments can be labor intensive due to the myriad of possible pediatric outcomes in trauma-exposed youth. PTSD, depression, anxiety, externalizing distress, and substance abuse (Cicchetti & Banny, 2014) are just some of the responses service providers may see in traumatized youth. Similarly, contextualizing these symptoms, along with school and other indices of behavioral functioning, is needed for an accurate knowledge of a student's trauma response. Therefore, having a broad knowledge of pediatric psychopathology, as well as the student's ecology and culturally-relevant background (de Arellano & Danielson, 2008), is vital to conducting a thorough trauma assessment.

Over the past 20 years, several instruments have been developed to assess traumatic events and responses in youth. Many of these measures can be located through the National Child Traumatic Stress Network (www.nctsn.org). The Juvenile Victimization Questionnaire (Finkelhor, Ormrod, Turner, & Hamby, 2005) is a comprehensive screening tool for assessing some of the more common forms of trauma experienced by children and adolescents (e.g., conventional crime, child maltreatment, witnessing and indirect victimization). Meanwhile, the UCLA-PTSD-RI (Rodriguez, Steinberg, & Pynoos, 1999) is a valid and reliable assessment of PTSD symptoms in a diverse group of children and adolescents (Hawkins & Radcliffe, 2006) that is widely used by clinicians and researchers alike.

It is important to note that some psychological distress reported during a trauma assessment may be independent from the CTE itself. In other words, it is important to determine (as best as possible) whether symptoms (a) predate the CTE, (b) were exacerbated by the CTE, or (c) emerged following the CTE. Caregivers, or longstanding service providers, are instrumental in helping to determine if a student's presentation is part of the trauma response and thus warrants trauma-focused treatment. School-based mental health counselors seeking to address trauma-related distress may identify empirically based treatments for trauma-exposed youth through a range of publically available resources, such as the California Evidence-Based Clearinghouse for Child Welfare (CEBCCW; http://www.cebc4cw.org/) and SAMHSA's National Registry of Evidence-based Programs and Practices (NREPP; http://www.nrepp.samhsa.gov/). Trauma-Focused Cognitive Behavioral Therapy (TF-CBT; Cohen et al., 2012) is a therapeutic approach that is "well-supported and efficacious" (Chaffin & Friedrich, 2004), with over 10 RCTs supporting its efficacy and successful implementations in school settings (Little, Akin-Little, & Gutierrez, 2009).

Finally, consistent with a positive psychology approach to clinical assessment (Wright & Lopez, 2009), it is important to assess for strengths in the student, caregiver, and community. While our chapter focused on negative outcomes from traumatic experiences, it is important to understand that resilience (a return to the child's previous level of functioning; Masten, 2001) is the norm, and posttraumatic growth (in which students demonstrate strengths or qualities beyond pre-trauma levels; Kilmer, 2006) is the reality for many. Importantly, resilience and posttraumatic growth can be fostered by understanding intrapersonal and interpersonal resources of support. In a review of the literature, Meyerson, Grant, Carter, and Kilmer (2011) found that social support, religiosity, reflective rumination, and pre-existing mental health were important predictors of positive outcomes following a traumatic event in youth. Identifying variables related to resilience and posttraumatic growth during the assessment process can help school mental health providers promote positive outcomes even in the wake of potentially traumatic events.

Conclusions and Future Directions

Traumatic events are common during childhood and adolescence, and school mental health providers need to have the clinical acumen to identify impacted youth. However, this is a significant challenge because, as reviewed above, trauma responses are extremely diverse. Internalizing (e.g., withdrawn behavior, negative affect, depressogenic cognitions) as well as externalizing (e.g., disruptive behavior, peer conflict, risky behavior and decision-making) symptoms are both common correlates of CTEs. As these responses are diverse and cut across trauma type (e.g., maltreatment compared to community violence), there is not a specific profile school personnel can look for that would suggest a specific traumatic event may have taken place. Instead, school personnel should be aware that behaviors and/or symptoms observed within the school context may be associated with trauma exposure, and specific procedures should be in place to assess and support those students. Changes in behavior, or developmentally inappropriate behaviors (e.g., sexually acting out at a young age) in general may warrant heightened awareness that a given child or adolescent may be living in an adverse family environment or have recently experienced some other traumatic event.

Although the negative consequences resulting from CTEs are widespread, the emerging findings concerning neglect are particularly alarming (see Boyce & Maholmes, 2013). As neglected youth may present as more withdrawn compared to non-neglected youth, these children may be more difficult to identify compared to other traumatized children who may be more externalizing in their behavior (Wilson, Norris, Shi, & Rack, 2008). Furthermore, as neglect is an omission of a behavior, rather than a commission of a behavior, it may be more difficult for school personnel to observe and assess for neglect as opposed to other forms of CTEs that may have been experienced by the community (e.g., school violence) or left a visible mark (e.g., a bruise from physical abuse). While neglect screeners do exist (e.g., the Childhood Trauma Questionnaire; Bernstein et al., 2003), a standard, neglect-specific semi-structured interview has yet to emerge and is needed. School personnel are likely to be among the only supportive adults that neglected youth interact with on a daily basis and, therefore, they can serve an especially important role for these youth.

Whether a CTE impacts an individual student (e.g., physical abuse) or an entire community (e.g., natural disaster), school providers can play a key role in supporting these youth and preventing further exposure. It is conservatively estimated that fewer than 1 in 5 students who have experienced a CTE receive the necessary clinical services (Overstreet & Mathews, 2011). Given that teachers and other school providers may be in a unique position to observe functional impairment in school engagement and academic performance, they can help connect impacted youth. Being aware of the possible consequences and how to assess for CTEs represents key steps towards bridging this need. Disclosures of CTEs to any school provider need to be taken seriously and reported to mental health services immediately. Likewise, disruptions in behavior or the emergence of emotional distress in students may be an indicator of CTEs. With the integration of empirically based trauma treatment in school settings (e.g., Little et al., 2009), trauma disclosures can now be translated into targeted services that can address students' mental health needs and improve their overall school performance.

Take-Home Points

- Childhood traumatic events (CTEs) are common and can impair youth across functional domains.
- Developmental cascade models have been instrumental in demonstrating how maltreatment experiences are associated with psychological distress and academic impairment, and they highlight key developmental stages for intervention.
- Community violence is pervasive in urban settings and even indirect exposure can have a profound impact on student's behavior in school.
- Trauma assessments need to (1) be inclusive of the traumatic event and psychological distress, (2) assess for any previous CTEs, (3) include an assessment of intrapersonal and interpersonal strengths, and (4) be behaviorally specific.

Resources

- Screening tools for trauma related responses (e.g., PTSD) can be located at the National Child Traumatic Stress Network website (http://www.nctsn.org/).
- School-based mental health counselors seeking to address trauma-related distress may identify empirically based treatments for trauma-exposed youth through a range of publically available resources, such as the California Evidence-Based Clearinghouse for Child Welfare (CEBCCW; http://www.cebc4cw.org/) and SAMHSA's National Registry of Evidence-based Programs and Practices (NREPP; http://www.nrepp.samhsa.gov/).

References

Bernstein, D.P., Stein, J.A., Newcomb, M.D., Walker, E., Pogge, D., Ahluvalia, T., . . . Zule, W. (2003). Development and validation of a brief screening version of the Childhood Trauma Questionnaire. *Child Abuse & Neglect, 27*, 169–190.

Bonanno, G.A., Brewin, C.R., Kaniasty, K., & La Greca, A.M. (2010). Weighing the costs of disaster consequences, risks, and resilience in individuals, families, and communities. *Psychological Science in the Public Interest, 11*, 1–49.

Boyce, C.A., & Maholmes, V. (2013). Attention to the neglected prospects for research on child neglect for the next decade. *Child Maltreatment, 18*, 65–68.

Buka, S.L., Stichick, T.L., Birdthisle, I., & Earls, F.J. (2001). Youth exposure to violence: Prevalance, risks, and consequences. *American Journal of Orthopsychiatry, 71*, 298–310.

Chaffin, M., & Friedrich, B. (2004). Evidence-based treatments in child abuse and neglect. *Children and Youth Services Review, 26*, 1097–1113.

Cicchetti, D., & Banny, A. (2014). A developmental psychopathology perspective on child maltreatment. In M. Lewis & K.D. Rudolph (Eds.), *Handbook of developmental psychopathology* (pp. 723–741). New York: Springer.

Cicchetti, D., & Rogosch, F.A. (1996). Equifinality and multifinality in developmental psychopathology. *Development and Psychopathology, 8*, 597–600.

Cloitre, M., Stolbach, B.C., Herman, J.L., Kolk, B.V.D., Pynoos, R., Wang, J., & Petkova, E. (2009). A developmental approach to complex PTSD: Childhood and adult cumulative trauma as predictors of symptom complexity. *Journal of Traumatic Stress, 22*, 399–408.

Cohen, J.A., Mannarino, A.P., & Deblinger, E. (2012). *Trauma-focused CBT for children and adolescents: Treatment applications*. New York: The Guilford Press.

Cohen, J.R., Danielson, C.K., Adams, Z.W., & Ruggiero, K.J. (2014). Distress tolerance, social support, and trauma symptoms: A longitudinal examination of internalizing and externalizing symptoms in youth. *Journal of Traumatic Stress*. Under review.

Costello, E.J., Erkanli, A., Fairbank, J.A., & Angold, A. (2002). The prevalence of potentially traumatic events in childhood and adolescence. *Journal of Traumatic Stress, 15*, 99–112.

Crozier, J.C., & Barth, R.P. (2005). Cognitive and academic functioning in maltreated children. *Children & Schools, 27*, 197–206.

Cullerton-Sen, C., Cassidy, A.R., Murray-Close, D., Cicchetti, D., Crick, N.R., & Rogosch, F.A. (2008). Childhood maltreatment and the development of relational and physical aggression: The importance of a gender-informed approach. *Child Development, 79*, 1736–1751.

Daniels, J.A., & Bradley, M.C. (2011). *Preventing lethal school violence*. New York: Springer.

de Arellano, M.A., & Danielson, C.K. (2008). Assessment of trauma history and trauma-related problems in ethnic minority child populations: An INFORMED approach. *Cognitive & Behavioral Practice, 15*, 53–67.

Egeland, B., Yates, T., Appleyard, K., & Van Dulmen, M. (2002). The long-term consequences of maltreatment in the early years: A developmental pathway model to antisocial behavior. *Children's services: Social policy, research, and practice, 5*, 249–260.

Erickson, M.F., & Egeland, B. (2011). Child neglect. In J.E.B. Myers (Ed.), *The APSAC handbook on child maltreatment* (3rd ed., pp. 103–124). Sage: Los Angeles, CA.

Fantuzzo, J.W., Perlman, S.M., & Dobbins, E.K. (2011). Types and timing of child maltreatment and early school success: A population-based investigation. *Children and Youth Services Review, 33*, 1404–1411.

Finkelhor, D., Ormrod, R.K., & Turner, H.A. (2007). Poly-victimization: A neglected component in child victimization. *Child Abuse & Neglect, 31*, 7–26.

Finkelhor, D., Ormrod, R.K., Turner, H., & Hamby, S.L. (2005). The victimization of children and youth: A comprehensive, national survey. *Child Maltreatment, 10*, 5–25.

Finkelhor, D., Turner, H., Hamby, S., & Ormrod, R. (2014). Polyvictimization: Children's exposure to multiple types of violence, crime, and abuse. *Free Inquiry in Creative Sociology, 39*, 24–34.

Finkelhor, D., Turner, H.A., Shattuck, A., & Hamby, S.L. (2013). Violence, crime, and abuse exposure in a national sample of children and youth: An update. *JAMA pediatrics, 167*, 614–621.

Flynn, R.J., Ghazal, H., Legault, L., Vandermeulen, G., & Petrick, S. (2004). Use of population measures and norms to identify resilient outcomes in young people in care: An exploratory study. *Child & Family Social Work, 9*, 65–79.

Ford, J.D., Chapman, J., Mack, J.M., & Pearson, G. (2006). Pathways from traumatic child victimization to delinquency: Implications for juvenile and permanency court proceedings and decisions. *Juvenile and Family Court Journal, 57*, 13–26.

Fowler, P.J., Tompsett, C.J., Braciszewski, J.M., Jacques-Tiura, A.J., & Baltes, B.B. (2009). Community violence: A meta-analysis on the effect of exposure and mental health outcomes of children and adolescents. *Development and Psychopathology, 21*, 227–259.

Furr, J.M., Comer, J.S., Edmunds, J.M., & Kendall, P.C. (2010). Disasters and youth: a meta-analytic examination of posttraumatic stress. *Journal of Consulting and Clinical Psychology, 78*, 765.

Guerra, N.G., Rowell Huesmann, L., & Spindler, A. (2003). Community violence exposure, social cognition, and aggression among urban elementary school children. *Child Development, 74*, 1561–1576.

Haw, C., Hawton, K., Niedzwiedz, C., & Platt, S. (2013). Suicide clusters: A review of risk factors and mechanisms. *Suicide and Life-Threatening Behavior, 43*, 97–108.

Hawkins, S.S., & Radcliffe, J. (2006). Current measures of PTSD for children and adolescents. *Journal of Pediatric Psychology, 31*, 420–430.

Howe, T.R., & Parke, R.D. (2001). Friendship quality and sociometric status: between-group differences and links to loneliness in severely abused and nonabused children. *Child Abuse & Neglect, 25*, 585–606.

Janosz, M., Archambault, I., Pagani, L.S., Pascal, S., Morin, A.J., & Bowen, F. (2008). Are there detrimental effects of witnessing school violence in early adolescence? *Journal of Adolescent Health, 43*, 600–608.

Jaycox, L.H., Stein, B.D., & Wong, M. (2014). School intervention related to school and community violence. *Child and Adolescent Psychiatric Clinics of North America, 23*, 281–293.

Kaplow, J.B., Howell, K.H., & Layne, C.M. (2014). Do circumstances of the death matter? Identifying socioenvironmental risks for grief:-Related psychopathology in bereaved youth. *Journal of Traumatic Stress, 27*, 42–49.

Kaplow, J.B., & Widom, C.S. (2007). Age of onset of child maltreatment predicts long-term mental health outcomes. *Journal of Abnormal Psychology, 116*, 176.

Katz, K.B. (1992). Communication problems in maltreated children: A tutorial. *Journal of Childhood Communication Disorders, 14*, 147–163.

Kazemian, L., Widom, C.S., & Farrington, D.P. (2011). A prospective examination of the relationship between childhood neglect and juvenile delinquency in the Cambridge study in delinquent development. *International Journal of Youth and Family Studies, 2*, 65–82.

Kilmer, R.P. (2006). Reslience and posttraumatic growth in children. In L.G. Calhoun & R.G. Tedeschi (Eds.), *Handbook of postrruamtic growth: Research & practice* (pp. 264–288). Mahwah, NJ: Lawrence Erlbaum Associates.

Kim, J., & Cicchetti, D. (2006). Longitudinal trajectories of self-system processes and depressive symptoms among maltreated and nonmaltreated children. *Child Development, 77*, 624–639.

Kisiel, C., Conradi, L., Fehrenbach, T., Torgersen, E., & Briggs, E.C. (2014). Assessing the effects of trauma in children and adolescents in practice settings. *Child and Adolescent Psychiatric Clinics of North America, 23*, 223–242.

Kolk, B.A.V.K. (2005). Developmental trauma disorder. *Psychiatric Annals, 35*, 401–408.

Kurtz, P.D., Gaudin, Jr., J.M., Wodarski, J.S., & Howing, P.T. (1993). Maltreatment and the school-aged child: School performance consequences. *Child Abuse & Neglect, 17*, 581–589.

La Greca, A.M., Silverman, W.K., Lai, B., & Jaccard, J. (2010). Hurricane-related exposure experiences and stressors, other life events, and social support: Concurrent and prospective impact on children's persistent posttraumatic stress symptoms. *Journal of Consulting and Clinical Psychology, 78*, 794.

Lai, B.S., La Greca, A.M., Auslander, B.A., & Short, M.B. (2013). Children's symptoms of posttraumatic stress and depression after a natural disaster: Comorbidity and risk factors. *Journal of Affective Disorders, 146*, 71–78.

Lansford, J.E., Dodge, K.A., Pettit, G.S., Bates, J.E., Crozier, J., & Kaplow, J. (2002). A 12-year prospective study of the long-term effects of early child physical maltreatment on psychological, behavioral, and academic problems in adolescence. *Archives of Pediatrics & Adolescent Medicine, 156*, 824–830.

Leiter, J. (2007). School performance trajectories after the advent of reported maltreatment. *Children and Youth Services Review, 29*, 363–382.

Little, S.G., Akin-Little, A., & Gutierrez, G. (2009). Children and traumatic events: Therapeutic techniques for psychologists working in the schools. *Psychology in the Schools, 46*, 199–205.

Lopez-Castroman, J., Jaussent, I., Béziat, S., Guillaume, S., Baca-Garcia, E., Olié, E., & Courtet, P. (2014). Posttraumatic Stress Disorder following childhood abuse increases the severity of suicide attempts. *Journal of Affective Disorders, 170*, 7–14.

Low, S., & Espelage, D. (2014). Conduits from community violence exposure to peer aggression and victimization: Contributions of parental monitoring, impulsivity, and deviancy. *Journal of Counseling Psychology, 61*, 221.

Manly, J.T., Kim, J.E., Rogosch, F.A., & Cicchetti, D. (2001). Dimensions of child maltreatment and children's adjustment: Contributions of developmental timing and subtype. *Development and psychopathology, 13*, 759–782.

Margolin, G., & Vickerman, K. (2007). Posttraumatic stress in children and adolescents exposed to family violence: I. Overview and issues. *Professional Psychology: Research and Practice, 1*, 613–619. doi: 10.1037/2160-4096.1.S.63

Martel, M.M., Pierce, L., Nigg, J.T., Jester, J.M., Adams, K., Puttler, L.I., . . . & Zucker, R.A. (2009). Temperament pathways to childhood disruptive behavior and adolescent substance abuse: Testing a cascade model. *Journal of Abnormal Child Psychology, 37*, 363–373.

Masten, A.S. (2001). Ordinary magic: Resilience processes in development. *American Psychologist, 56*(3), 227.

Masten, A.S., & Cicchetti, D. (2010). Developmental cascades. *Development and Psychopathology, 22*(03), 491–495.

Mathews, T., Dempsey, M., & Overstreet, S. (2009). Effects of exposure to community violence on school functioning: The mediating role of posttraumatic stress symptoms. *Behaviour Research and Therapy, 47*(7), 586–591.

Meyerson, D.A., Grant, K.E., Carter, J.S., & Kilmer, R.P. (2011). Posttraumatic growth among children and adolescents: A systematic review. *Clinical Psychology Review, 31*(6), 949–964.

Miller, M., Flynn, R.J., & Vandermeulen, G. (2008). *Looking after children in Ontario: Good parenting, good outcomes: Ontario provincial report (Year Six)*. Reports for 0–4, 5–9, 10–15, and 16–20 year olds. Ottawa: Centre for Research on Educational and Community Services, University of Ottawa.

Moreno-Manso, J.M., García-Baamonde, M.E., Alonso, M.B., & Barona, E.G. (2010). Pragmatic language development and educational style in neglected children. *Children and Youth Services Review, 32*, 1028–1034.

Nanni, V., Uher, R., & Danese, A. (2012). Childhood maltreatment predicts unfavorable course of illness and treatment outcome in depression: A meta-analysis. *American Journal of Psychiatry, 169*(2), 141–151.

Neiman, S., & DeVoe, J.F. (2009). Crime, violence, discipline, and safety in U.S. public schools: Findings from the school survey on crime and safety: 2007–08. Washington, DC: National Center for Education Statistics, Institute of Education Sciences, U.S. Department of Education.

Neumayer, E., & Barthel, F. (2011). Normalizing economic loss from natural disasters: A global analysis. *Global Environmental Change, 21*(1), 13–24.

Nikulina, V., Widom, C.S., & Czaja, S. (2011). The role of childhood neglect and childhood poverty in predicting mental health, academic achievement and crime in adulthood. *American Journal of Community Psychology, 48*, 309–321.

Overstreet, S., & Mathews, T. (2011). Challenges associated with exposure to chronic trauma: Using a public health framework to foster resilient outcomes among youth. *Psychology in the Schools, 48*(7), 738–754.

Resnick, H.S., Kilpatrick, D.G., Dansky, B.S., Saunders, B.E., & Best, C.L. (1993). Prevalence of civilian trauma and posttraumatic stress disorder in a representative national sample of women. *Journal of Consulting and Clinical Psychology, 61*(6), 984.

Robinson, J., Cox, G., Malone, A., Williamson, M., Baldwin, G., Fletcher, K., & O'Brien, M. (2013). A systematic review of school-based interventions aimed at preventing, treating, and responding to suicide-related behavior in young people. *Crisis: The Journal of Crisis Intervention and Suicide Prevention, 34*(3), 164.

Rodriguez, N., Steinberg, A., & Pynoos, R.S. (1999). UCLA PTSD index for DSM IV instrument information: Child version, parent version, adolescent version. *UCLA Trauma Psychiatry Services*. Los Angeles, CA.

Rogosch, F.A., Oshri, A., & Cicchetti, D. (2010). From child maltreatment to adolescent cannabis abuse and dependence: A developmental cascade model. *Development and Psychopathology*, *22*(04), 883–897.

Romano, E., Babchishin, L., Marquis, R., & Fréchette, S. (2014). Childhood maltreatment and educational outcomes. *Trauma, Violence, & Abuse*, doi: 1524838014537908

Rosenfield, D., Jouriles, E.N., McDonald, R., & Mueller, V. (2014). Interparental conflict, community violence, and child problems: Making sense of counterintuitive findings. *American Journal of Orthopsychiatry*, *84*(3), 275.

Saunders, B.E., & Adams, Z.W. (2014). Epidemiology of traumatic experiences in childhood. *Child and adolescent psychiatric clinics of North America*, *23*(2), 167–184.

Schell, T.L., Marshall, G.N., & Jaycox, L.H. (2004). All symptoms are not created equal: The prominent role of hyperarousal in the natural course of posttraumatic psychological distress. *Journal of Abnormal Psychology*, *113*(2), 189.

Selby, E.A., Anestis, M.D., Bender, T.W., & Joiner, Jr., T.E. (2009). An exploration of the emotional cascade model in borderline personality disorder. *Journal of Abnormal Psychology*, *118*(2), 375.

Shields, A., & Cicchetti, D. (2001). Parental maltreatment and emotion dysregulation as risk factors for bullying and victimization in middle childhood. *Journal of Clinical Child Psychology*, *30*, 349–363.

Slade, E.P., & Wissow, L.S. (2007). The influence of childhood maltreatment on adolescents' academic performance. *Economics of Education Review*, *26*(5), 604–614.

Snyder, H.N., & Sickmund, M. (2006). Juvenile offenders and victims: 2006 national report. *Office of Juvenile Justice and Delinquency Prevention*.

Stein, M., Schork, N., & Gelernter, J. (2007). Gene-by-environment (serotonin transporter and childhood maltreatment) interaction for anxiety sensitivity, an intermediate phenotype for anxiety disorders. *Neuropsychopharmacology*, *33*, 312–319. doi: 10.1038/sj.npp.1301422

Tiesl, M., & Cicchetti, D. (2008). Physical abuse, cognitive and emotional process, and aggressive/disruptive behavior problems. *Social Development*, *16*, 1–23.

Voisin, D.R., Neilands, T.B., & Hunnicutt, S. (2011). Mechanisms linking violence exposure and school engagement among African American adolescents: Examining the roles of psychological problem behaviors and gender. *American Journal of Orthopsychiatry*, *81*(1), 61–71.

Weems, C.F., Taylor, L.K., Costa, N.M., Marks, A.B., Romano, D.M., Verrett, S.L., & Brown, D.M. (2009). Effect of a school-based test anxiety intervention in ethnic minority youth exposed to Hurricane Katrina. *Journal of Applied Developmental Psychology*, *30*, 218–226.

Wilson, S.R., Norris, A.M., Shi, X., & Rack, J.J. (2008). Comparing physically abused, neglected, and nonmaltreated children during interactions with their parents: A meta-analysis of observational studies. *Communication Monographs*, 77, 540–575.

Wright, B.A., & Lopez, S.J. (2009). Widening the diagnostic focus. In C.R. Snyder & S.J. Lopez (Eds.), *Handbook of positive psychology* (pp. 26–44). New York, NY/London, UK: Oxford University Press.

15

FAMILY ENGAGEMENT IN SCHOOL-BASED MENTAL HEALTH

Eleanor Castine, Sean Flanagan, and Kimberly A.S. Howard

Family involvement in schools has been found to support improvements in academic achievement and to facilitate positive socio-emotional outcomes for children and youth in the areas of emotion regulation, social competence, and mental health (Hoagwood et al., 2010). A child's mental health is inextricably linked to the family, school, and community systems in which she/he is embedded (Hill & Craft, 2003). Thus, creating collaborative partnerships across these systems can increase the efficacy of intervention efforts (Reinke, Splett, Robeson, & Offutt, 2009) and has become a fundamental principle that most school-based mental health professionals (SBMHPs) are encouraged to practice (Quinn & Lee, 2007).

Why Is Family Engagement Important?

SBMHPs are motivated to involve caregivers in the mental health treatment of their children beyond the informed consent stage for several reasons (Motes, Melton, Simmons, & Pumariega, 1999). Family engagement in school-based mental health treatment has been found to a) be a predictor of mental health outcomes, b) positively impact families as well as the students, and c) facilitate the treatment process for SBHMPs.

Predictors of Mental Health Outcomes

Research indicates that even with partial family engagement in mental health treatment, children experience symptom reduction (Jaycox et al., 2010). Schools and families historically have been disconnected contexts for children (Bryan & Henry, 2008), resulting in inconsistent rules, boundaries, and expectations for children's behavior between these two systems. This can lead to confusion and stress for children (Eppler & Weir, 2009). Establishing and supporting a connection between school and home is crucial to building congruency across these two settings in a child's life. Engaging families may be especially relevant when working with racial and ethnic minority populations as well as low-income families (Davis, Ressler, Schwartz, Stephens, & Bradley, 2009). The centrality of family and involvement of extended family members is not only an important cultural value within these groups, but close family connections have also been shown to be a protective factor from emotional disturbance for children (Pumariega & Vance, 1999).

Impact on Families

Families, too, benefit from involvement in their children's mental health treatment. Hoagwood and colleagues (2010) found that family engagement in their children's treatment resulted in a reduction in stress, improved mental health and well-being, increased self-efficacy, higher perceived social support, and stronger treatment engagement for parents and caregivers. Collectively, these factors only serve to improve overall family functioning. Further, creating relationships with families gives opportunities for all voices to be heard, facilitating better understanding of the family by SBMHPs and increasing the likelihood of effective collaboration and healthy outcomes (Eppler & Weir, 2009). Engaging families in treatment allows for the process to be redefined such that it is one of shared power between the families and SBMHPs with mutual roles and responsibilities (Bryan & Henry, 2008).

Impact on Students

In a review of more than 50 studies, Henderson and Mapp (2002) found that family-school collaboration is related to better student attendance, improved behavior at home and school, and better social skills and adaptation to school. Further, involving families in the mental health treatment of their children allows parents/caregivers to modify any potentially problematic family management skills, particularly those that are predictive of poor mental health outcomes for children and youth (Hammen, Rudolph, Weisz, Rao, & Burge, 1999; Stormshak, Bierman, McMahon, Lengua, & Conduct Problems Prevention Research Group, 2000).

Advantages for School-based Mental Health Professionals

Family involvement allows for a more comprehensive and accurate assessment of the child and his/her challenges. Further, a team approach to treatment reduces the risk of burnout among educators and other service providers, allowing them to remain engaged, empathic, and effective over time (Cohen & Cohen, 2000).

Finally, such an approach involves and models an emphasis on mutual respect and shared accountability for student outcomes, which supports positive outcomes for children across systems (Shapiro et al., 2010).

What Does Good Family Engagement Look Like?

Despite the clear importance of family engagement in school-based mental health treatment, fostering and sustaining such engagement remains a challenge (Santiago et al., 2013). Success in building positive relations with families begins with a clear conceptualization of "family engagement." Hoagwood and colleagues (2010) conceptualize "engagement" as involving four processes: initial engagement, collaboration, support, and empowerment. These processes are distinct, yet interrelated, and may be differentially useful at different times and for different purposes.

Initial engagement is the process of forming a connection with families at the beginning of treatment that sets the tone for the course of treatment. Making engagement a priority at the outset helps to create a safe space in which families can be open about their concerns, goals, and expectations. This process also involves ongoing and open dialogue about helpful treatment strategies and methods to maximize treatment success for the child.

Next, **collaboration** between the family and the SBMHP requires both parties to appreciate the expertise that one another possesses and is marked by shared power and decision-making. SBMHPs can encourage collaboration by conveying care and concern to the family, engaging the family members as partners in treatment, and developing joint goals for their work. The essence of treatment shifts when family members feel like equal partners in the process, often resulting in greater sharing of information by family members, increased flexibility and availability for meetings, and a better understanding of the limits of SBMHPs (DeChillo, 1993).

Third, the process of **support** entails providing family members with helpful information, encouragement, and reinforcement. When a child is struggling, it can be incredibly draining for the entire family. Families may feel helpless or lack the knowledge and awareness of resources available to them. SBMHPs endeavor to ensure that a family is given the support required to address their child's needs. There are various types of support that SBMHPs can offer families, including informational, instructional, emotional, instrumental, and advocacy (Hoagwood et al., 2010). Informational support, for example, could involve educating a family about the course of mental illness, its impact, and different treatment options.

Finally, **empowerment** involves "helping families become active and competent agents of change" (Hoagwood, 2005, p. 701). SBMHPs can reduce perceived barriers to treatment, enhancing families' abilities to participate in services (Hoagwood et al., 2010). SBMHPs can increase a family's sense of empowerment by giving them the power to make decisions, a range of treatment options, and access to resources (Chamberlain, 1996). Ultimately, empowerment can foster a sense of hope and the ability to persist in the face of challenge (Hoagwood et al., 2010).

Factors That Predict Family Engagement

School-based mental health professionals (SBMHPs) can use the concepts of initial engagement, collaboration, support, and empowerment to improve the frequency and quality of family engagement. Hoover-Dempsey and Sandler (HDS; 2005) developed a model of parent involvement in schools detailing the school- and family-based factors that influence the variety and frequency of parent involvement in the academic achievement of their children (Walker, Shenker, & Hoover-Dempsey, 2010). We have adapted the HDS factors in content and structure according to extant literature on family engagement in school-based mental health services, and have redefined them as being reflective of *Family Factors* or *School Factors*.

Family Factors

According to the HDS model, three categories of parent-factors can influence family involvement in schools: a) personal motivators, b) families' perceptions of invitations to be involved, and c) life context variables. Each of these categories will be discussed in relation to school-based mental health services, with examples provided to illustrate cultural considerations.

Personal motivators. Motivation for engagement is shaped by the social context in which a parent develops and exists. Current and past experiences with education, mental health, and family systems, for example, inform parents' **role construction** and **self-efficacy** regarding engagement in school-based mental health services. **Role construction** refers to a parent's beliefs about what one should do in relation to the child's school-based mental health services. In conceptualizing the role that one should play, parents consider the purpose and scope of their participation in school-based mental health services (Hoover-Dempsey & Sandler, 2005). **Self-efficacy** on the other hand, is a parent's belief about whether he/she is competent to engage in their child's treatment and the extent to which engagement will have a positive influence (Bandura, 1993). In short, parents are influenced by their beliefs about the role that they can play in their child's treatment and how well they believe they can play it. Parents' beliefs about their role and their personal efficacy can be influenced by broad past experiences with school engagement or previous attempts to engage specifically with school-based mental health services (Hoover-Dempsey & Sandler, 2005). Furthermore, interventions that are perceived as threatening family stability or a challenge to parental authority may result in ineffective treatment or premature termination (Erickson & Al-Timimi, 2001). Finally, parents may feel considerable guilt regarding the nature of their child's mental health difficulties. As such, parents may be reluctant to engage insofar as they perceive themselves to have contributed negatively to the child's mental health issues (Lieberman, Van Horn, & Ippen, 2005). Helping parents build positive beliefs around their *role construction* and *self-efficacy* is crucial for engaging parents in school-based mental health services.

Family perceptions of welcome. The family's decision to engage in school-based mental health services depends largely on whether they feel invited by the school community, SBMHPs, and the child (Cohen, Linker, & Stutts, 2006). Schools can feel very unwelcoming to family members (Weist et al., 2009). Lack of school outreach or negative attitudes from staff, teachers, custodians, and SBMHPs can deter parents from engaging in school-based mental health services. For example, staff and administrators may have competing priorities and believe that giving control and resources to parents will diminish their ability to achieve alternative educational goals of the school (Cohen et al., 2006). Culturally speaking, language barriers or perceptions of discrimination also influence the extent to which parents feel invited by schools to engage (Gopalan, Burton, McKay, & Rosenzweig, 2008). Feeling welcome can be especially important for certain populations, such as families of undocumented status who may have legal concerns and fear the educational and health systems (Toppelberg, Hollinshead, Collins, & Nieto-Castañon, 2013). Parents' decisions to engage with schools are shaped by specific invitations from SBMHPs, such as requests for parents to support treatment at home or attend a family session at school (Hoover-Dempsey & Sandler, 2005). Perhaps most importantly, engagement is determined by parent perceptions of specific invitations from the child.

Life context variables. In addition to the aforementioned potential barriers, family engagement in school-based services may be further complicated by variables such as (a) family level of functioning (b) family resources, and (c) culture (Cohen et al., 2006). Parent/caregiver level of functioning is an important predictor of engagement (Hoover-Dempsey & Sandler, 2005). Physical or mental health disabilities may constrain parents' abilities to participate in school engagement. For example, parents might have mental health issues or trauma of their own that reduces their likelihood and ability to engage in the child's treatment (Lieberman et al., 2005; Snell-Johns, Mendez, & Smith, 2004). Further, families' perceptions of the unique skills, knowledge, and psychological mindedness of their family may influence engagement. For instance, families that lack an understanding of the school organization and culture are less likely to engage with school-based mental health services (Johnson, Pugach, & Hawkins, 2004). Despite school requests for family engagement, if families believe that their knowledge or skills are inadequate, they may be less likely to take action.

Engagement is largely dependent upon the family's resources. Limited time, lack of childcare, transportation, and scheduling flexibility due to work or other family obligations may create challenges for engaging families (Davis et al., 2009; Stevens, Kelleher, Ward-Estes, & Hayes, 2006). Furthermore, these resources are largely affected by systemic factors and may disproportionately affect specific populations, including single parents; ethnic minorities; and those experiencing poverty, inadequate health insurance, social stigma, and neighborhood disadvantage (Snell-Johns et al., 2004; Toppelberg et al., 2013). Ensuring that families are able to overcome barriers to treatment is particularly important because families from low income backgrounds and those with children with the greatest service needs have the lowest level of school participation (Park, Pullis, Reilly, & Townsend, 1994). Families with fewer resources and greater demands often find themselves confronted with the difficult choice between the much-needed economic gains of work and engaging in their children's mental health treatment (Eppler & Weir, 2009).

Further, culture plays a significant role in shaping a family's decision to collaborate with school personnel. Cultural beliefs shape parents' perceptions of services, treatment, and goals. For example, some caregivers may not appreciate the relevance of understanding a child's needs, the systems, and communication with SBMHPs (Toppelberg et al., 2013). Some cultures attribute great stigma to mental health issues and may not support engagement in these services. Moreover, parents and SBMHPs may have culturally divergent views on whether or not a child has a problem that requires services (De Los Reyes & Kazdin, 2005). In the event that families disagree with treatment goals, find little or no benefit to services, or perceive providers as judgmental, they are less likely to initiate or sustain engagement (Gross, Julion, & Fogg, 2001).

School Factors

While many factors related to parents and families undoubtedly influence the likelihood of family engagement, successful collaboration is affected by variables related to schools as well. Much like families, schools often have limited resources with which they can successfully engage families. Additionally, while families' decisions are shaped by beliefs and values, so too are the actions of schools as reflected in their service delivery model.

Limited resources. Schools are often constrained by available resources. They have limited ability to meet family needs, such as weekend or evening appointments, child care, and transportation (Santiago et al., 2013; Weist et al., 2009; Reinke et al., 2009;). These limitations lead to obvious logistical and communication challenges as SBMHPs have neither the time nor means to meet the growing need to engage families (Johnson et al., 2004). Yet, collaboration and engagement may actually be a more efficient and worthwhile approach to delivering services than current practices (Eppler & Weir, 2009).

Governing model of service delivery. The model used to guide mental health service delivery greatly influences SBMPHs engagement with families. For example, SBMHPs face competing responsibilities placed on them by schools, as educational and fiscal priorities often dictate treatment options (Eppler & Weir, 2009; Reinke et al., 2009; Santiago et al., 2013). Moreover, most SBMHPs are guided by an individual model of services and may lack formal training and knowledge around engaging parents (Reinke et al., 2009). Thus, while resources may be available to effectively engage parents/caregivers, the clinical decision to do so ultimately lies with SBMPHs and the schools in which they operate.

Recommendations for Engaging Families

While family engagement is by no means easy, school-based mental health treatment can greatly reduce barriers to care. Families and Schools Together (FAST), existing in seven countries and all 50 states, serves as an example of an evidence-based treatment that effectively engages parents to build a bridge between home and school (McDonald, Billingham, Conrad, Morgan, Nina, & Payton, 1997). It is essential that SBMHPs take the necessary steps to promote family engagement at the same time that they minimize barriers for engagement in treatment. The HDS model of parental involvement in schools can be adapted to provide a framework for engaging families in their child's school-based mental health services.

Incorporate Family and Parent Values, Goals, Expectations, and Aspirations

As mentioned above, good family engagement emphasizes the importance of the initial relationship-building with families as active family involvement positively influences health outcomes (Johnson et al., 2004). Creating a shared vision and identifying goals for treatment facilitates the development of individualized plans of care to meet the unique needs of the child and family (Pumariega & Vance, 1999). Developing a shared vision requires families to be included as equal participants, co-defining the child's problem and deciding upon the best and most culturally responsive approach to treatment across school and home contexts (Cohen et al., 2006). Families bring unique value to the collaborative treatment team, providing invaluable knowledge about the child, his/her strengths and needs, and the child's treatment history.

Parents' values, expectations, and aspirations can be assessed through initial interviews or meetings, fostering a collaborative tone for future engagement (Stormshak, Fosco, & Dishion, 2010). Maintaining a family's level of engagement requires the collaborative team to continually evaluate progress toward goals and the collaborative process itself (Cohen et al., 2006). This is perhaps best accomplished by inviting all members of the team to provide feedback on the treatment and the process of working together, particularly since informants often disagree in their reports of a child's behavior (Grills & Ollendick, 2003; De Los Reyes & Kazdin, 2005; Cohen et al., 2006). Continued assessment ensures that families' values, expectations, and aspirations are successfully incorporated into their child's treatment.

Successful collaboration often employs a strengths-based approach to partnership in which strengths and assets of the collaborating parties are emphasized rather than deficits or problems (Cohen et al., 2006; Shapiro, DuPaul, Barnabas, Benson & Slay, 2010). A strengths-based approach focuses on characteristics that foster collaboration across home and school systems and build trusting, long-term relationships between school and families. Creating the foundation for the strengths-based approach begins with identifying the key collaborative parties (e.g. family, SBMHP) and the positive assets that each can contribute to the current task (Cohen et al., 2006).

Effective Communication Among Families, SBMHPs, and Schools

Engaging families through a collaborative process of school-based mental health treatment is contingent upon the frequency and quality of communication between parents and schools. Effective communication is marked by mutual respect, careful listening, and school responsiveness to families' questions, ideas, suggestions, and concerns (Hoover-Dempsey & Sandler, 2005). Effective communication can be supported by collaborative decisions to formalize roles and development of a partnership language. Families must come to know the role that they play within the collaboration and how it differs from the role of other parties. In addition, the establishment of a partnership language can ensure successful communication across parties. Key terms, concepts, and processes are redefined to form a common language that is understood and used by all (Cohen et al., 2006).

The quantity of communication should also be considered in addition to the quality. Families often desire more communication, information, and personal contact with clinicians than they are provided (Santiago et al., 2013). Methods of communication should be selected according to the resources available to the family. For example, among low-income populations, SBMHPs may need to make an extra effort by calling instead of mailing a letter. The quantity and nature of communication that occurs between families and schools should be agreed upon early and evaluated continually to ensure that communication meets the needs of both parties.

Create a Welcoming School Culture and Effective Staff

Encourage voluntary involvement in school community. Schools can demonstrate the desire for parent engagement broadly through providing opportunities for parents to volunteer in the school community. Creating roles for parents to volunteer within the school-based mental health services system, such as a parent liaison role, can lead to better mental health outcomes for youth and higher engagement among parents (Kutash et al., 2013).

Establish a culture of trust. Schools can promote parent engagement by establishing and demonstrating a culture of trust between the school and families.

Parents that have trust in the school and/or SBMHP may be more likely to encourage their child to engage in treatment (Santiago et al., 2013). Establishing trust, personal connections, and communicating empathy can be modeled by all staff within the school (Santiago et al., 2013), and begins with the expression of mutual respect for the knowledge and expertise that all parties, including parents, have regarding the child (Minke & Anderson, 2005; Cohen et al., 2006; Reinke et al., 2009). Avoiding an "us versus them" mentality is imperative for creating a welcoming environment for parents.

Have highly qualified staff. Creating a welcoming culture that promotes parent engagement often relies on developing a highly qualified staff. While all members of the collaborative partnership play a significant role, SBMHPs are perhaps best situated to promote family engagement. SBMHPs have an in-depth understanding of the stressors, needs, strengths, and characteristics associated with various mental health disorders. Moreover, they are familiar with the language, culture, and systems of the schools and community in which they work (Cohen et al., 2006). SBMHPs should strive to shape school-based mental health service delivery models by designing processes that fully engage families as partners. SBMHPs can encourage SBMHPs in training (e.g., social work interns, school counseling interns) and other school staff (e.g., teachers, administrators, secretarial and maintenance staff) to join in establishing the collaborative partnership with families.

Family Engagement in Activities at School

Family engagement can take many forms, including participation in parent training. Parent training is typically conducted in groups and can be led by SBMHPs or parents themselves. Peer-to-peer program models are often led by parents who have successfully navigated the school-based service delivery model and have received some training around helping other parents engage in their child's treatment (Kutash et al., 2013). Such groups focus on a range of goals and have been associated with many promising outcomes. For example, parent groups have focused on broad community level goals, such as reducing the stigma and isolation associated with mental health problems (Kutash et al., 2013). They can equip parents with the skills to implement interventions at home (Rones & Hoagwood, 2000) and are associated with increased access to mental health services, increased parental empowerment (Elliot, Koroloff, Koren, & Friesen, 1998), increased perceived social support (Ireys & Sakwa, 2006), as well as decreases in disruptive behavior and substance abuse among youth (Maughan, Christiansen, Jenson, Olympia, & Clark, 2005). Parent groups may be most impactful when they are structured to meet the particular developmental and mental health needs of the children (Rones & Hoagwood, 2000). For example, elementary groups might focus on behavior management strategies while groups for parents of older youth might focus on the prevention of substance use or on issues of developmental maturation (Rones & Hoagwood, 2000).

Family Engagement in Activities at Home

Parent training groups can provide parents with opportunities to learn skills and techniques for use at home with their children. These practices might include a daily check-in with the child about his/her day, mood, and any school-based services received that day. Families can assist the child in practicing coping skills, monitoring and reviewing therapy homework, and ensuring medication is taken consistently and properly. Through frequent high-quality communication with SBMHPs, parents can provide valuable information about the child's functioning, progress, and challenges at home. SBMHPs can engage parents in more formal evaluation of the treatment process by administering child and family assessments that parents can complete at home (Stormshak, et al., 2010). Family assessment is a valuable tool and has been identified as a best-practice for collecting data that can be used by schools to determine the efficacy of their work with families (Eppler & Weir, 2009). Whether trained by SBMHPs or through peer-to-peer models, families' implementation of interventions at home can provide continuity of care between children's environments in addition to empowering parents as valuable members of their child's treatment process.

Conclusion

In sum, family engagement in school-based mental health treatments supports positive outcomes for children and youth. SBMHPs can use the processes of initial engagement, collaboration, support, and empowerment to successfully partner with families in the treatment process. By addressing both the family-based and school-based factors that can serve to facilitate or hinder family involvement, SBMHPs increase the likelihood that productive and effective family-school collaborations are established.

Take-Home Points

- Engaging families in school-based mental health treatment predicts mental health outcomes, positively impacts families and students, and facilitates the treatment process for SBMHPs.
- Successful family engagement by SBMHPs is marked by initial engagement, collaboration, support, and empowerment.
- Family factors, including personal motivators, families' perceptions of invitations to be involved, and life context variables, in conjunction with school factors, such as limited resources and the governing model of service delivery, can greatly influence family engagement.
- To promote family engagement, it is recommended that SBMHPs focus on establishing a shared vision and goals for treatment, effective communication, the creation of a welcoming school culture, and increasing parent engagement in activities at school as well as at home.

Resources

- Families and Schools Together (FAST): http://familiesandschools.org

References

Bandura, A. (1993). Perceived self-efficacy in cognitive development and functioning. *Educational Psychologist, 28*(2), 117–148.

Bryan, J., & Henry, L. (2008). Strengths-based partnerships: A school-family-community partnership approach to empowering students. *Professional School Counseling, 12*(2), 149–156.

Chamberlain, P. (1996). Intensified foster care: Multilevel treatment for adolescents with conduct disorders in out-of-home care. In E.D. Hibbs & P.S. Jensen (Eds.), *Psychosocial treatments for child and adolescent disorders: Empirically based strategies for clinical practice* (pp. 475–495). Washington, DC: American Psychological Association.

Cohen, R., & Cohen, J. (2000). *Chiseled in sand: Perspectives on change in human services organization*. Belmont, CA: Wadsworth.

Cohen, R., Linker, J.A., & Stutts, L. (2006). Working together: Lessons learned from school, family, and community collaborations. *Psychology in the Schools, 43*(4), 419–428.

Davis, R.G., Ressler, K.J., Schwartz, A.C., Stephens, K.J., & Bradley, R.G. (2009). Treatment barriers for low-income, urban African Americans with undiagnosed posttraumatic stress disorder. *Journal of Traumatic Stress, 21*(2), 218–222.

DeChillo, N. (1993). Collaboration between social workers and families of patients with mental illness. *Families in Society, 74*, 104–115.

De Los Reyes, A., & Kazdin, A.E. (2005). Informant discrepancies in the assessment of childhood psychopathology: A critical review, theoretical framework, and recommendations for further study. *Psychological Bulletin, 131*(4), 483–509.

Elliot, D.J., Koroloff, N., Koren, P.D., & Friesen, B. (1998). Improving access to children's mental health services: The family associate approach. In M.H. Epstein, K. Kutash, & A.J. Duchnowski (Eds.), *Outcomes for children and youth with emotional disorders and their families: Programs and evaluation best practices* (pp. 581–609). Austin, TX: Pro-Ed.

Eppler, C., & Weir, S. (2009). Family assessment in K–12 settings: Understanding family systems to provide effective, collaborative services. *Psychology in the Schools, 46*(6), 501–514.

Erickson, C.D., & Al-Timimi, N.R. (2001). Providing mental health services to Arab Americans: Recommendations and considerations. *Cultural Diversity and Ethnic Minority Psychology, 7*, 308–327.

Gopalan, G., Burton, G., McKay, M.M., & Rosenzweig, J.M. (2008). Achieving school-family collaboration for children with emotional or behavioral disorders. In J.M. Rosenzweig & E.M. Brennan (Eds.), *Work, life, and the mental health system of care: A guide for professionals supporting families of children with emotional or behavioral disorders* (pp. 201–237). Baltimore: Paul H. Brookes.

Grills, A.E., & Ollendick, T.H. (2003). Multiple informant agreement and the Anxiety Disorders Interview Schedule for Parents and Children. *Journal of the American Academy of Child and Adolescent Psychiatry, 42*, 30–40.

Gross, D., Julion, W., & Fogg, L. (2001). What motivates participation and drop-out among low-income urban families of color in a prevention intervention? *Family Relations, 50*, 246–254.

Hammen, C., Rudolph, K., Weisz, J., Rao, U., & Burge, D. (1999). The context of depression in clinic-referred youth: Neglected areas in treatment. *Journal of the American Academy of Child & Adolescent Psychiatry, 38*(1), 64–71.

Henderson, A.T., & Mapp, K.L. (2002). *A new wave of evidence: The impact of school, family and community connections on student achievement.* Austin, TX: National Center for Family and Community Connections with Schools, Southwest Educational Development Laboratory.

Hill, N.E., & Craft, S.A. (2003). Parent-school involvement and school performance: Mediated pathways among socioeconomically comparable African American and Euro-American families. *Journal of Educational Psychology, 95*(1), 74–83.

Hoagwood, K.E. (2005). Family-based services in children's mental health: A research review and synthesis. *Journal of Child Psychology and Psychology, 46*(7), 690–713.

Hoagwood, K.E., Cavaleri, M.A., Olin, S.S., Burns, B.J., Slaton, E., Gruttadaro, D., & Hughes, R. (2010). Family support in children's mental health: A review and synthesis. *Clinical Child and Family Psychology Review, 13*(1), 1–45.

Hoover-Dempsey, K.V., & Sandler, H.M. (2005). The social context of parental involvement: A path to enhanced achievement: Final performance report for OERI Grant # R305T010673. Nashville, TN: Vanderbilt University. Retrieved from http://www.vanderbilt.edu/peabody/family-school/Reports.html

Ireys, H.T., & Sakwa, D. (2006). Building family-to-family support programs: Rationale, goals, and challenges. *Focal Point, 20*(1), 10–14.

Jaycox, L.H., Cohen, J.A., Mannarino, A.P., Walker, D.W., Langley, A.K., Gegenheimer, K.L., . . . Schonlau, M. (2010). Children's mental health care following Hurricane Katrina: A field trial of trauma-focused psychotherapies. *Journal of Traumatic Stress, 23*, 223–231.

Johnson, L.J., Pugach, M.C., & Hawkins, A. (2004). School-family collaboration: A partnership. *Focus on Exceptional Children, 36*(5), 1–12.

Kutash, K., Garraza, L.G., Ferron, J.M., Duchnowski, A.J., Walrath, C., & Green, A.L. (2013). The relationship between family education and support services and parent and child outcomes over time. *Journal of Emotional and Behavioral Disorders, 21*(4), 264–276.

Lieberman, A.F., Van Horn, P., & Ippen, C.G. (2005). Toward evidence-based treatment: Child-parent psychotherapy with preschoolers exposed to marital violence. *Journal of the American Academy of Child and Adolescent Psychiatry, 44*(12), 1241–1248.

Maughan, D.R., Christiansen, E., Jenson, W.R., Olympia, D., & Clark, E. (2005). Behavioral parent training as a treatment for externalizing behaviors and disruptive behavior disorders: A meta-analysis. *School Psychology Review, 34*(3), 267–286.

McDonald, L., Billingham, S., Conrad, P., Morgan, A., Nina O., & Payton, E. (1997). Families and Schools Together (FAST): Integrating community development with clinical strategy. *Families in Society, 78*(2), 140–155.

Minke, K.M., & Anderson, K.J. (2005). Family-school collaboration and positive behavior support. *Journal of Positive Behavior Interventions, 7*, 181–185.

Motes, P.S., Melton, G., Simmons, W.E.W., & Pumariega, A. (1999). Ecologically oriented school-based mental health services: Implications for service system reform. *Psychology in the Schools, 36*(5), 391–401.

Park, E.K., Pullis, M., Reilly, T.F., & Townsend, B.L. (1994). Cultural biases in the identification of students with behavioral disorders. In R.L. Peterson & S. Ishii-Jordan (Eds.), *Multicultural issues in the education of students with behavior disorders.* Cambridge, MA: Brookline Books.

Pumariega, A.J., & Vance, H.R. (1999). School-based mental health services: The foundation of systems of care for children's mental health. *Psychology in the Schools, 36*(5), 371–378.

Quinn, K.P., & Lee, V. (2007). The wraparound approach for students with emotional and behavioral disorders: Opportunities for school psychologists. *Psychology in the Schools, 44*(1), 101–111.

Reinke, W.M., Splett, J.D., Robeson, E.N., & Offutt, C.A. (2009). Combining school and family interventions for the prevention and early intervention of disruptive behavior problems in children: A public health perspective. *Psychology in the Schools, 46*(1), 33–43.

Rones, M., & Hoagwood, K. (2000). School-based mental health services: A research review. *Clinical Child and Family Psychology Review, 3*(4), 223–241.

Santiago, C.D., Pears, G., Bawjea, S., Vona, P., Tang, J., & Kataoka, S.H. (2013). Engaging parents in evidence-based treatments in schools: Community perspectives from implementing CBITS. *School Mental Health, 5*, 209–220.

Shapiro, E.S., DuPaul, G.J., Barnabas, E., Benson, J.L., & Slay, P.M. (2010). Facilitating school, family, and community partnerships: Enhancing student mental health: An overview of the special series. *School Mental Health, 2*, 45–51.

Snell-Johns, J., Mendez, J.L., & Smith, B.H. (2004). Evidence-based solutions for overcoming access barriers, decreasing attrition, and promoting change with underserved families. *Journal of Family Psychology, 18*(1), 19–35.

Stevens, J., Kelleher, K.J., Ward-Estes, J., & Hayes, J. (2006). Perceived barriers to treatment and psychotherapy attendance in child community mental health centers. *Community Mental Health Journal, 42*(5), 449–458.

Stormshak, E.A., Bierman, K.L., McMahon, R.J., Lengua, L., & Conduct Problems Prevention Research Group. (2000). Parenting practices and child disruptive behavior problems in early elementary school. *Journal of Clinical Child Psychology, 29*, 17–29.

Stormshak, E.A., Fosco, G.M., & Dishion, T.J. (2010). Implementing interventions with families in schools to increase youth school engagement: The Family Check-Up model. *School Mental Health, 2*(2), 82–92.

Toppelberg, C.O., Hollinshead, M.O., Collins, B.A., & Nieto-Castañon, A. (2013). Cross-sectional study of unmet mental health need in 5- to 7-year old Latino children in the United States: Do teachers and parents make a difference in service utilization? *School Mental Health, 5*, 59–69.

Walker, J.M.T., Shenker, S.S., & Hoover-Dempsey, K.V. (2010). Why do parents become involved in their children's education? Implications for school counselors. *Professional School Counseling, 14*(1), 28–41.

Weist, M., Lever, N., Stephan, S., Youngstrom, E., Moore, E., Harrison, B., . . . Stiegler, K. (2009). Formative evaluation of a framework for high quality evidence-based services in school mental health. *School Mental Health, 1*, 196–211.

16

UNIVERSAL PREVENTION TO SUPPORT CHILDREN'S MENTAL HEALTH IN SCHOOLS

Keith C. Herman, Wendy M. Reinke, Aaron M. Thompson, and Reuben Faloughi

As documented in chapters throughout this book, many promising and well-established interventions have been developed for treating even the most burdensome and debilitating mental health problems experienced by youth. Two overlapping realities, however, can interfere with the success of these interventions: (1) schools and communities rarely have enough resources to identify and provide intensive services for the large number of youth who experience severe emotional and behavioral problems; and (2) many youth who would benefit from early interventions to reduce risk go unnoticed and do not receive any services at all (see Herman, Merrell, Reinke, & Tucker, 2004; Reinke, Herman, & Tucker, 2006). It is exciting to have strategies that can help individuals overcome mental health problems. Without a broader approach, however, individual or group interventions will not impact the population health or reduce the incidence or prevalence of these conditions (Biglan, 1995).

A public health approach provides a framework for influencing population health outcomes (Reinke et al., 2006). Although elements of a public health framework applied to children's mental health—including the idea of conceptualizing health promotion, prevention, and treatment along a continuum—have appeared in several prominent reports (National Research Council & Institute of Medicine [NRC & IOM], 2000, 2009; National Research Council, Institute of

---

Authors' Note: Preparation of this manuscript was supported in part by the Institute of Education Sciences, U.S. Department of Education, through Grants R305A100342, R305A130375 (PI: Wendy Reinke) and R305A130143 (PI: Keith Herman) awarded to the University of Missouri. The opinions expressed are those of the authors and do not represent views of the Institute or the U.S. Department of Education.

Medicine, & Committee on Evaluation of Children's Health, 2004), the application of fully integrated models remains challenging. In particular, universal approaches to mental health promotion and prevention are often foreign to mental health providers who have been trained to deliver services to individuals or small groups.

In this chapter, we define universal prevention and situate it within a public health perspective. Next, we describe how this approach fits along a continuum of supports for students, ranging from minimal to intensive services, and show how this framework not only can reduce the number of students who will need intensive supports but also can help identify those most in need. We then describe examples of universal prevention models in school settings. We conclude with a discussion of barriers to universal prevention, potential solutions, and future directions.

Definitions and Rationale

The NRC and the IOM (2009) have been at the forefront of efforts to define prevention-related activities related to mental health. Modern definitions of prevention situate it along a continuum of activities ranging from prevention to treatment and maintenance. Prevention includes three levels characterized by increasing intensity of interventions: (1) universal prevention, which includes services or strategies delivered to an entire population without regard to risk status; (2) selective prevention, which targets specific subgroups based on the presence of an identified risk factor for the disease or outcome of interest; and (3) indicated prevention, which is delivered to persons showing early signs or symptoms that do not yet meet the threshold for a given disease or disorder (Stormont, Reinke, & Herman, 2010). The modern language of prevention parallels and replaces prior public health terminology, which included primary, secondary, and tertiary prevention.

Tiered response models have been developed in educational settings that align with these different prevention activities. Some fundamental premises of the tiered prevention approach to youth mental health problems are that (a) all children can benefit from universal supports; (b) risk of progressing to more intensive service needs can be mitigated for many children by intervening earlier with less intensive supports; and (c) non-response to less intensive services can help better identify those most in need of intensive support (Thompson, Reinke, & Herman, in press).

In particular, a universal prevention framework offers strategies to reduce negative emotional and behavioral outcomes and increase positive mental health outcomes for entire populations (NRC & IOM, 2009). The goal of universal prevention is to address risk and protective factors that contribute to problems on a wide-scale basis, regardless of an individual's risk in the population (Split, Koot, & van Lier 2013). Universal prevention activities often involve indirect services and activities such as consultation to promote healthy social environments, system-wide interventions and supports, media campaigns, or public policy changes.

Key Etiological Dimensions and Best Practices for Assessment and Identification

A key element of successful application of tiered response models is to have efficient data collection systems to monitor and quickly identify risk and protective factors as well as youth response to each tier of services. In public health and epidemiology, surveillance systems provide continuous, systematic data streams to help plan, implement, and evaluate practices (World Health Organization, 2012).

Effective and efficient surveillance systems require the identification of intended outcomes along with corresponding etiological factors. Social-ecological models provide a useful framework for considering risk and protective factors associated with negative mental health outcomes. These models suggest that emotional and behavior problems are embedded within a series of interacting contextual systems from broader social and cultural systems (schools, families) to internal, within-person systems (perceptual, biological, and genetic) (Herman et al., 2004). Traditionally, interventions to alleviate social emotional symptoms have focused on systems that are more proximal to the individual, particularly within person factors, by providing skills training, individual therapy, or medication. Research has shown that successful youth interventions often require intervention in family and/or school subsystems that surround the youth. These interventions are grounded in the assumption and empirical research showing that youth problems often originate in pathogenic interactions with their social environment, and thus altering these environments can alleviate symptoms (Biglan, Flay, Embry, & Sandler, 2012). A corollary of this assumption, also supported by evidence, is that altering these social environments prior to the emergence of youth symptoms can prevent problems from emerging in the first place (NRC & IOM, 2009).

A recent theory of nurturing environments proffered by Biglan and colleagues (2012) suggests that most major youth social and emotional problems can be traced at least in part to problems in several environmental circumstances: toxic life events, limited opportunities to learn and practice prosocial behaviors and socioemotional skills, and an absence of adult supervision (Biglan et al., 2012). In contrast, nurturing environments help optimize child mental health outcomes by reducing toxic life events such as maltreatment and physical injury; providing abundant opportunities to learn self-awareness, emotional regulation, and social skills; and monitoring youth activities. Biglan and colleagues provided an extensive review of literature, including a series of comprehensive reviews by the NRC and IOM (2000, 2009; National Research Council, Institute of Medicine, & Committee on Evaluation of Children's Health, 2004), to support the importance of each nurturing environment domain.

A surveillance approach to identifying risk and protective factors involves continual monitoring of these environmental risk and protective conditions as well as student behaviors and outcomes indicative of unsuccessful/successful adaptation. In school settings, nurturing environments requires that students feel safe, physically and socially; expectations are clear and reasonable; students receive higher rates of more positive than negative attention from adults and peers; consequences are predictable; and social, emotional, and academic competence is fostered. Continuous data streams can be gathered from systematized school records (e.g., office discipline referrals [ODRs], absences), student surveys/ratings, and teacher reports (McIntosh, Reinke, & Herman, 2010). These data are then used to guide local decision-making about student responsiveness to intervention (e.g., a student with two or more ODRs may be identified as not responding to universal school-wide supports and in need of selective or intensive supports) and areas for school improvement.

Examples of Universal Supports in Schools

Schools are composed of multiple subsystems that can be the targets of universal supports. These include school-wide or setting-specific systems (playground, classroom, cafeteria, hallways, etc.). Rather than reviewing all available universal interventions that have been developed for each of these systems, here we describe exemplars within three key school subsystems: school-wide, classroom, and student level supports.

School-Wide

School-wide programs and practices attempt to alter broad social systems and interactions so that they are more nurturing and likely to promote positive youth development and reduce known ecological risk factors. School disorder characterized by punitive adult interactions, limited adult supervision, aversive peer interactions, and little support for student autonomy and competence undermines youth development and contributes to risk for most major youth mental disorders (Herman et al., 2004; Reinke & Herman, 2002). For instance, although externalizing disorders can often be traced to early pathogenic family environments, school environments often exacerbate and accelerate these early symptoms (Reinke & Herman, 2002). Patterson, Reid, and Dishion's (1992) cascade model includes a clear description of how the coercive cycle at home that contributes to early-onset antisocial behaviors often is repeated with adult interactions at schools (Reinke & Herman, 2002). Additionally, children with these behaviors are often rejected by peers at school, encounter learning difficulties, and ultimately drift to delinquent peer groups that further reinforce their behavior patterns. In a similar manner, school environments can contribute to risk for internalizing symptoms and disorders (Herman et al., 2004).

School-Wide Positive Behavior Interventions and Supports (SW-PBIS) is a proactive behavior support model that was developed two decades ago as a public health approach to reduce school disorder and promote positive student outcomes (Sugai, Horner, & Gresham, 2002). Since 2000, nearly 20,000 schools in the U.S. have implemented SW-PBIS; in ten states, over 40% of the schools use the approach (Horner, 2013). On a school-wide level, PBIS involves having school staff develop clear behavior expectations in all school settings; model, teach, and practice the expectations; provide higher rates of positive than negative attention for meeting these expectations; and collect systematic data of behavior infractions, including type, location, time, and other descriptors. The data is then used by school-based teams to make decisions about how well the universal system is working and to identify areas of improvement (e.g., if a high number of infractions occurs on the playground, the team would decide how to reduce the problem perhaps by reteaching expectations, increasing adult supervision, and/or increasing positive attention rates). Additionally, tools are used to monitor the fidelity of implementation of PBIS to ensure desired outcomes are achieved.

SW-PBIS is not a curriculum or a packaged program. Rather it is a framework and set of strategies for building more nurturing environments in schools. Abundant resources are available for schools to use as they implement the model, including national and state technical assistance centers and web resources (see www.pbis.org).

Many single subject studies have supported the impact of PBIS in reducing problem behaviors in school specific settings (see Reinke et al., 2006). More recently, two randomized trials have augmented these smaller, less rigorous studies and found that PBIS implementation was associated with improvements in school safety, academic achievement, positive student behaviors, and school climate compared to control schools (Bradshaw, Koth, Thornton, & Leaf, 2009; Bradshaw, Mitchell, & Leaf, 2010; Bradshaw, Waasdorp, & Leaf, 2012; Horner et al., 2009).

Classroom

Several examples of classroom-level universal prevention exist. The exemplars in this category train all teachers, regardless of risk, to provide effective classroom behavior management skills. Much like the literature showing the importance of effective parent behavior management skills in fostering healthy child adaptation, much research shows the value of clear and predictable, supportive classroom environments in supporting positive youth development (Biglan et al., 2012).

The Good Behavior Game (GBG) is probably the most studied intervention in this category. Developed in the late 1960s by a classroom teacher, the GBG is a method for inhibiting student misbehavior in the classroom through social contingencies (Barrish, Saunders, & Wolf, 1969). Through a systematic process, teachers are taught to play the game by dividing the class into teams, setting clear expectations, tracking behavior infractions, and rewarding the team with the fewest infractions at intervals throughout the day. The research base in support of the GBG is fairly remarkable, with over 20 randomized trials supporting its effects in reducing adverse youth outcomes, prompting Embry (2002) to label it as a "behavior vaccine." More recent studies have shown that the protective social and emotional health benefits from even a single year exposure to GBG during first grade persist into adulthood (Bradshaw, Zmuda, Kellam, & Ialongo, 2009; Kellam et al., 2008; Kellam, Wang, et al., 2014). Moreover, early exposure to GBG improves educational outcomes through high school, including persistence and graduation (Bradshaw et al., 2009).

The Incredible Years Teacher Classroom Management (IY TCM) program, a companion to the well-established IY Parent program, is a 5- or 6-session full day workshop training series with ongoing coaching that is focused on equipping elementary school teachers with effective classroom management skills. Skills are organized in a hierarchy, conceptualized as a Teaching Pyramid; foundation skills and practices focus on establishing positive relationships with youth and clear expectations. Higher level skills, which are used less frequently, include strategies for setting limits consistently (e.g., ignoring, logical consequences, time out) (see http://incredibleyears.com/download/resources/teacher-pgrm/teacher-program-pyramid.pdf). A unique aspect of IY TCM is that teachers are also taught how to "coach" social and emotional skills in school settings by modeling the skills and prompting their use throughout the school day. Several prior RCTs in Head Start and elementary school settings have shown the promise of IY TCM in fostering effective teaching practices, including increasing teachers' use of praise, consistent consequence, and nurturing interactions (Webster-Stratton et al., 2010; see Webster-Stratton & Herman, 2010). Additionally, children in IY TCM classrooms have been found to have lower levels of observed aggression and higher rates of on-task and prosocial behaviors. Additionally, Raver and colleagues (2008) found strong effects (d = 0.52 to 0.89) for a multi-component intervention that included the IY TT program on classroom climate and teacher behaviors in 36 Head Start classrooms (602 students). All of these prior studies, however, had included IY TCM has part of a multi-component intervention (combined with IY Parent, or IY Child, or both).

A more recent trial with 105 classrooms and 1818 students in kindergarten through 3rd grade from a large urban district randomly assigned to IY TCM or to a wait-list control showed moderate effects on teacher behaviors (e.g., use of proactive teaching strategies) and small but significant effects on student prosocial behaviors and self-regulation skills (Reinke, Herman, & Dong, 2014). Small effects are expected from universal preventive interventions given that they are delivered to entire populations without regard to risk (i.e., many individuals would not develop disorders even without the intervention); yet even very small effects on a population level can result in dramatic improvements in public health outcomes (NRC & IOM, 2009). Additional training programs using similar practices and procedures have been developed for secondary teachers (Allen et al., 2011; Herman et al., 2014).

Universal Student Skill Training

More direct universal services to promote student mental health involve explicit social and coping skills instruction. Many such programs have been developed for application in schools. Most of these programs involve teaching specific skills in the classroom (either by the teacher or other school professionals) and are tailored to different developmental levels.

Social emotional programs—such Promoting Alternative Thinking Strategies (PATHS) and Second Step (SS)—build upon decades of prevention and intervention science guided by the integration of social learning and information processing theories and applied research findings from studies on empathy training and cognitive behavioral interventions. Considered "best practices" by the U.S. Centers for Disease Control (Thornton, Craft, Dahlberg, Lynch, & Baer, 2000) and "evidence-based programs" by the Substance Abuse and Mental Health Services Administration's National Registry of Evidence-Based Programs and Practices (http://www.nrepp.samhsa.gov/AboutNREPP.aspx), programs such as PATHS and SS include comprehensive curricula that aim to improve short-term social and emotional knowledge and skills.

PATHS (Greenberg, Kusche, Cook, & Quamma, 1995) targets youth ages 0–5 (preschool) and 6–12 (elementary) using over 100 lessons designed to be delivered by classroom teachers to increase emotional self and social awareness, self-management, problem solving, and relationship skills. SS (Frey, Hirschstein, et al., 2005; Grossman et al., 1997) is a classroom-based social emotional skills program for youth ages 4–14 (preschool through middle school) that aims to increase social competencies and prosocial behaviors while reducing impulsive and aggressive behaviors. Though there are many social emotional programs to choose from, these programs target similar mechanisms and are widely believed to be effective at influencing a host of desirable student and school level outcomes. Though mixed, the balance of findings from early efficacy trials, systematic reviews, and more recent effectiveness studies in both the U.S. and Europe suggest that social emotional learning programs produce mild but significant effects for important student and school level outcomes (Durlak et al., 2011; Heckman & Kautz, 2012).

Integrating Universal With Selective and Indicated Interventions

Recent efforts have focused on integrating prevention programs to determine whether even stronger effects can be observed in combination than with a single program. Potential advantages of integrated approaches include the possibility of targeting multiple risk factors simultaneously, the potential for additive or even synergistic effects, and the broader reach of combined approaches (Domitrovich et al., 2010).

Domitrovich and colleagues described two types of integrated models: horizontal and vertical. Horizontal approaches combine preventative interventions within the same risk category, such as integrating two or more universal prevention approaches. Vertical integration combines preventive interventions across risk levels, such as combining a universal and a selective intervention. Several examples of vertical integrations exist, including school-wide programs like SW-PBIS, which have tiered response frameworks embedded within them. Common selective components in SW-PBIS include small group social skills training and a group level program called the Behavior Education program or Check-in Check-out system; indicated interventions in the PBIS framework usually involve functional behavior assessment and behavior support planning (Reinke et al., 2006).

Barriers and Solutions

While universal school-based prevention approaches hold great promise for preventing negative mental health outcomes among youth on a large scale, several barriers can impede implementation in school settings. The first set of barriers concern the practical implementation challenges that any type of social, behavioral, and educational intervention needs to consider. In schools, these barriers include limited resources and infrastructure to support high quality implementation over time (Gottfredson & Gottfredson, 2002). Most public schools in the U.S. have many competing education priorities and pressures, often changing year to year, which limit the attention and resources that can be given to social and emotional health promotion and mental health prevention (Botvin, 2004).

Notably, the pragmatic concerns of solving immediate crises in school settings often leaves little time for considering alternative approaches that are needed to prevent the problems in the first place. A major tenet of a universal prevention approach is that if the prevalence of a targeted behavior (such as office discipline referrals in schools) in a given setting (school, neighborhood, community, etc.) exceeds 15–20%, resources are better devoted to bolstering the universal supports in that setting rather than to providing more direct clinical services (Reinke et al., 2006). The rationale is that such high rates of disorder indicate that most youth in that setting are not being provided the basic supports needed for successful adaptation. Communities and schools will simply never have enough resources to provide intensive supports and direct services to such large segments of their population. Higher quality universal prevention strategies reduces the number of youth in need of services.

Unfortunately, most school professionals are unaware of the evidence-based prevention practices or the guiding conceptual framework described in this chapter (Stormont, Reinke, & Herman, 2011). Although most school professionals identify managing student disruptive behaviors as the most challenging aspect of their jobs (Reinke, Stormont, Herman, Puri, & Goel, 2011), the reactive and punitive approaches that many schools use to address these problems usually makes them worse (Atkins et al., 2002). Thus, disseminating training and skill development in evidence-based preventive approaches is a key priority to overcoming many of these implementation barriers. Incorporating training in these methods in teacher preparation and school psychology/counseling/child clinical training programs is an obvious first step. Additionally, national and statewide technical assistance models that have been used to support the widespread dissemination of SW-PBIS (see www.pbis.org) provide an instructive model for how to reach the legions of school professionals currently in practice.

Tools for monitoring the fidelity of implementation to these practices are also needed. Again, SW-PBIS serves as a model in this regard. The School-wide Evaluation Tool (SET) is a measure that is used to monitor fidelity and give feedback to schools about the quality of implementation (Horner et al., 2004). Research supports the use of this tool and includes minimal benchmarks that align with desired impacts on student behaviors. Additionally, tools and strategies for monitoring classroom level interventions like IY TCM have been developed and described (Webster-Stratton et al., 2011).

A final barrier to consider pertains to cultural and professional ideologies that may conflict with a prevention-oriented approach (Shadish, 1984). Although the concept of prevention is intuitively appealing, commitment to actions that are necessary for prevention practices to occur requires a certain set of beliefs and values that may not align with individual or national identities. Investment in universal prevention activities often contradicts beliefs associated with individualistic cultural values such as self-determination and meritocracy (Gregory, 2001). Additionally, prevention activities may conflict with the professional identities of clinically oriented psychologists, counselors, and educators, many of whom have been trained to conceptualize pathology within individuals and deliver services to clients one person at a time rather than intervening in broader systems. Thus, widespread implementation of effective prevention practices requires confronting and altering aspects of these cultural or professional ideologies (see Herman et al., 2004).

Summary and Future Directions

The progress in preventing major mental health symptoms and syndromes provides much reason for optimism about the continued development of effective universal prevention practices. Innovations in system-level interventions and multi-tiered supports will continue to bolster efforts to impact population mental health (not just individuals). Future research will need to examine essential mechanisms of these models, particularly school-wide models, and examine their effects in reducing the incidence of disorders in addition to their known effects on symptoms.

Take-Home Points

- Without a public health approach, individual or group interventions will not impact the population health or reduce the incidence or prevalence of these conditions.

- A key element of successful application of universal prevention models is to have efficient data collection systems to monitor and quickly identify risk and protective factors as well as youth outcomes.
- A nurturing environment perspective is useful for understanding factors that foster or hinder youth development.
- Schools are composed of various subsystems, including school-wide, classroom, and individual student levels, that can be the target of universal prevention activities.
- A strong evidence base supports the success of universal prevention activities in schools to reduce problem behaviors and promote healthy student development.
- Successful adoption and widespread dissemination of universal prevention requires confronting conflicting cultural and professional ideologies, as well as providing necessary training to support high quality implementation.

Resources

- National Positive Behavior Interventions and Supports Technical Assistance Center: www.pbis.org
- Incredible Years: incredibleyears.com
- My Teaching Partner: http://www.mtpsecondary.net/
- CHAMPS: http://www.safeandcivilschools.com

References

Allen, J.P., Pianta, R.C., Gregory, A., Mikami, A.Y., & Lun, J. (2011). An interaction-based approach to enhancing secondary school instruction and student achievement. *Science, 333*(6045), 1034–1037.

Atkins, M.S., McKay, M.M., Frazier, S.L., Jakobsons, L.J., Arvanitis, P., Cunningham, T., . . . & Lambrecht, L. (2002). Suspensions and detentions in an urban, low-income school: Punishment or reward? *Journal of Abnormal Child Psychology, 30*(4), 361–371.

Barrish, H.H., Saunders, M., & Wolf, M.M. (1969). Good behavior game: Effects of individual contingencies for group consequences on disruptive behavior in a classroom. *Journal of Applied Behavior Analysis, 2*(2), 119–124.

Biglan, A. (1995). Translating what we know about the context of antisocial behavior into a lower prevalence of such behavior. *Journal of Applied Behavior Analysis, 28*, 479–492.

Biglan, A. (2001). Contextualism and the development of effective prevention practices. *Prevention Science, 5*, 15–21.

Biglan, A., Flay, B.R., Embry, D.D., & Sandler, I.N. (2012). The critical role of nurturing environments for promoting human well-being. *American Psychologist, 67*(4), 257.

Botvin, G.J. (2004). Advancing prevention science and practice: Challenges, critical issues, and future directions. *Prevention Science, 5*(1), 69–72.

Bradshaw, C.P., Koth, C.W., Thornton, L.A., & Leaf, P.J. (2009). Altering school climate through school-wide Positive Behavioral Interventions and Supports: Findings from a group-randomized effectiveness trial. *Prevention Science, 10*(2), 100–115.

Bradshaw, C.P., Mitchell, M.M., & Leaf, P.J. (2010). Examining the effects of schoolwide positive behavioral interventions and supports on student outcomes results from a randomized controlled effectiveness trial in elementary schools. *Journal of Positive Behavior Interventions, 12*(3), 133–148.

Bradshaw, C.P., Waasdorp, T.E., & Leaf, P.J. (2012). Effects of school-wide positive behavioral interventions and supports on child behavior problems. *Pediatrics, 130*(5), e1136–e1145.

Bradshaw, C.P., Zmuda, J.H., Kellam, S.G., & Ialongo, N.S. (2009). Longitudinal impact of two universal preventive interventions in first grade on educational outcomes in high school. *Journal of Educational Psychology, 101*(4), 926.

Domitrovich, C.E., Bradshaw, C.P., Greenberg, M.T., Embry, D., Poduska, J.M., & Ialongo, N.S. (2010). *Integrated models of school-based prevention: Logic and theory. Psychology in the Schools*, 47(1), 71–88.

Durlak, J.A., Weissberg, R.P., Dymnicki, A.B., Taylor, R.D., & Schellinger, K.B. (2011). The impact of enhancing students' social and emotional learning: A meta-analysis of school-based universal interventions. *Child Development, 82*(1), 405–432.

Embry, D.D. (2002). The Good Behavior Game: A best practice candidate as a universal behavioral vaccine. *Clinical Child and Family Psychology Review, 5*(4), 273–297.

Frey, K.S., Hirschstein, M.K., Snell, J.L., Edstrom, L.V.S., MacKenzie, E.P., & Broderick, C.J. (2005). Reducing playground bullying and supporting beliefs: An experimental trial of the steps to respect program. *Developmental Psychology, 41*(3), 479.

Greenberg, M.T., Kusche, C.A., Cook, E.T., & Quamma, J.P. (1995). Promoting emotional competence in school-aged children: The effects of the PATHS curriculum. *Developmental Psychopatholy*, 7, 117–117.

Gregory, R.J. (2001). The spirit and substance of community psychology: Reflections. *Journal of Community Psychology, 29*, 473–485.

Gottfredson, D.C., & Gottfredson, G.D. (2002). Quality of school-based prevention programs: Results from a national survey. *Journal of Research in Crime and Delinquency, 39*, 3–35.

Grossman, D.C., Neckerman, H.J., Koepsell, T.D., Liu, P.-Y., Asher, K.N., Beland, K., . . . Rivara, F.P. (1997). Effectiveness of a violence prevention curriculum among children in elementary school. *JAMA: the journal of the American Medical Association, 277*(20), 1605–1611.

Heckman, J.J., & Kautz, T. (2012). Hard evidence on soft skills. *Labour Economics, 19, 451–464.*

Herman, K.C., Merrell, K., Reinke, W.M., & Tucker, C.M. (2004). The role of school psychology in preventing and treating depression. *Psychology in the Schools, 41*, 763–775.

Herman, K.C., Reinke, W.M., Petree, M., Lewis, C., Colletta, A., & Faloughi, R. (2014). *Evaluation of a classroom management program for middle school students.* Poster presented at the 6th Annual Educational, School, & Counseling Psychology Conference, Columbia, MO.

Horner, R. (2013). *Moving PBIS forward with quality, equity, and efficiency*. Presentation at the Utah MTSS Conference.

Horner, R.H., Sugai, G., Smolkowski, K., Eber, L., Nakasato, J., Todd, A.W., & Esperanza, J. (2009). A randomized, wait-list controlled effectiveness trial assessing school-wide positive behavior support in elementary schools. *Journal of Positive Behavior Interventions, 11*(3), 133–144. doi: http://dx.doi.org/10.1177/1098300709332067

Horner, R.H., Todd, A.W., Lewis-Palmer, T., Irvin, L.K., Sugai, G., & Boland, J.B. (2004). The School-Wide Evaluation Tool (SET): A research instrument for assessing School-Wide Positive Behavior Support. *Journal of Positive Behavior Interventions, 6*(1), 3–12.

Institute of Medicine (IOM). (1994). *Reducing the risk for mental disorder: Frontiers of prevention intervention research.* Washington, DC: National Academies Press.

Kellam, S.G., Brown, C.H., Poduska, J.M., Ialongo, N.S., Wang, W., Toyinbo, P., . . . & Wilcox, H.C. (2008). Effects of a universal classroom behavior management program in first and second grades on young adult behavioral, psychiatric, and social outcomes. *Drug and Alcohol Dependence, 95,* S5–S28.

Kellam, S.G., Wang, W., Mackenzie, A.C., Brown, C.H., Ompad, D.C., Or, F., . . . & Windham, A. (2014). The impact of the Good Behavior Game, a universal classroom-based preventive intervention in first and second grades, on high-risk sexual behaviors and drug abuse and dependence disorders into young adulthood. *Prevention Science, 15*(1), 6–18.

McIntosh, K., Reinke, W., & Herman, K.C. (2010). School-wide analysis of data for social behavior problems: Assessing outcomes, selecting targets for intervention, and identifying need for support. In G.G. Peacock, R.A. Irvin, E.J. Daly, & K. Merrell (Eds.), *Practical handbook of school psychology: Effective practices for the 21st century.* New York: Guilford Press.

National Research Council & Institute of Medicine (NRC & IOM). (2000). *From neurons to neighborhoods: The science of early childhood development.* Committee on Integrating the Science of Early Childhood Development. Washington, DC: The National Academies Press.

National Research Council & Institute of Medicine (NRC & IOM). (2009). *Preventing mental, emotional, and behavioral disorders among young people: progress and possibilities.* Committee on Prevention of Mental Disorders and Substance Abuse Among Children, Youth, and Young Adults: Research Advances and Promising Interventions. Washington, DC: The National Academies Press.

National Research Council, Institute of Medicine, & Committee on Evaluation of Children's Health. (2004). *Children's health, the nation's wealth: Assessing and improving child health.* Washington, DC: The National Academies Press.

Patterson, G., Reid, J., & Dishion, T. (1992). *Antisocial boys.* Eugene, OR: Castalia Publishing Company.

Raver, C.C., Jones, S.M., Li-Grining, C.P., Metzger, M., Champion, K.M., & Sardin, L. (2008). Improving preschool classroom processes: Preliminary findings from a randomized trial implemented in Head Start settings. *Early Childhood Research Quarterly, 23*(1), 10–26.

Reinke, W.M., & Herman, K.C. (2002). Creating school environments that deter antisocial behaviors in youth. *Psychology in the Schools, 39,* 549–559.

Reinke, W.M., Herman, K.C., & Dong, N. (2014, March). A group randomized evaluation of the Incredible Years Teacher Training program. Paper presented as part of symposium entitled, *What can we learn through replication? The role of individual-level risk factors and implementation supports in the impact of social-emotional learning programs on student outcomes* at The Society for Research on Educational Effectiveness Annual Conference, Washington, DC.

Reinke, W.M., Herman, K.C., & Tucker, C.M. (2006). Building and sustaining communities that prevent mental disorders: Lessons from the field of special education. *Psychology in the Schools, 43,* 313–329.

Reinke, W., Stormont, M., Herman, K.C., Puri, R., & Goel, N. (2011). Supporting children's mental health in schools: Teacher perceptions of needs, roles, and barriers. *School Psychology Quarterly, 26,* 1–13.

Shadish, W.R. (1984). Policy research: Lessons from the implementation of deinstitutionalization. *American Psychologist, 39*, 725–738.

Split, J.L., Koot, J.M., van Lier, P.A.C. (2013). For whom does it work? Subgroup differences in the effects of a school-based universal prevention program. *Prevention Science, 14*, 479–488.

Sprick, R., Garrison, M., & Howard, L. (2009). *CHAMPS: A proactive and positive approach to classroom management* (2nd ed.). Eugene, OR: Pacific Northwest Publishing.

Stormont, M., Reinke, W.M., & Herman, K.C. (2010). Using prevention science to address mental health issues in schools. *Psychology in the Schools, 47*, 1–4.

Stormont, M., Reinke, W., & Herman, K.C. (2011). Teachers' knowledge of evidence-based interventions and available school resources for children with emotional or behavioral problems. *Journal of Behavioral Education, 20*, 138–147.

Sugai, G., Horner, R.H., & Gresham, F.M. (2002). Behaviorally effective school environments. In M.R. Shinn, H.M. Walker, & G. Stoner (Eds.), *Interventions for academic and behavior problems II: Preventive and remedial approaches* (pp. 315–350). Bethesda, MD: National Association of School Psychologists.

Taub, J. (2002). Evaluation of the Second Step violence prevention program at a rural elementary school. *School Psychology Review, 31*(2), 186–200.

Thompson, A.M., Reinke, W.M., & Herman, K.C. (in press). The value, practice, and evaluation of teaching social emotional learning to students with and without disabilities. In C.R. Massat, M.S. Kelly, & R. Constable (Eds.), *School social work: Practice, policy, and research* (8th ed.). New York: Oxford.

Thornton, T.N., Craft, C.A., Dahlberg, L.L., Lynch, B.S., & Baer, K. (2000). *Best Practices of Youth Violence Prevention: A Sourcebook for Community Action.*

Webster-Stratton, C., & Herman, K.C. (2010). Disseminating Incredible Years Series Early Intervention Programs: Integrating and sustaining services between school and home. *Psychology in the Schools, 47*, 36–54.

Webster-Stratton, C., & Reid, M.J. (2010). The Incredible Years Parents, Teachers and Child Training Series: A multifaceted treatment approach for young children with conduct problems. In J.R. Weisz & A.E. Kazdin (Eds.), *Evidence-based psychotherapies for children and adolescents* (2nd ed., pp. 194–210). New York, NY: Guilford Press.

Webster-Stratton, C., Reinke, W., Herman, K.C., Newcomer, L. (2011). The Incredible Years Teacher Training: The methods and principles that support fidelity of training delivery. *School Psychology Review, 40*, 509–529.

World Health Organization. (2012). *Public health surveillance.* Retrieved from http://www.who.int/topics/public_health_surveillance/en/

CONTRIBUTORS

Heidemarie Blumenthal, Ph.D., Assistant Professor, Director of the Teen Stress and Alcohol Research (Teen St.A.R.) Laboratory, University of North Texas Department of Psychology

Caroline L. Boxmeyer, Ph.D., Associate Professor, Department of Psychiatry and Behavioral Medicine, College of Community Health Sciences, The University of Alabama

Cheryl Buehler, Ph.D., Professor, Human Development and Family Studies, University of North Carolina Greensboro

Eleanor Castine, M.S., Doctoral student in Counseling Psychology, School of Education, Boston University

Renee M. Cloutier, B.A., Doctoral student in Experimental Psychology, University of Texas

Joseph R. Cohen, Ph.D., Post-doctoral Fellow, National Crime Victims Research and Treatment Center, Department of Psychiatry and Behavioral Sciences, Medical University of South Carolina

Cassandra L. Colbert, B.S., Doctoral student in Counseling Psychology, College of Education, University of Illinois at Urbana-Champaign

Carla Kmett Danielson, Ph.D., Associate Professor, National Crime Victims Research and Treatment Center, Department of Psychiatry and Behavioral Sciences, Medical University of South Carolina

Kimberly DeBoth, M.A., Doctoral student in School Psychology, Department of Educational Psychology, Ball State University

Dorothy L. Espelage, Ph.D., Gutgsell Professor, Child Development Division, College of Education, University of Illinois at Urbana-Champaign

Reuben Faloughi, B.S., Doctoral student in Counseling Psychology, Department of Educational, School, and Counseling Psychology, University of Missouri

Sean Flanagan, M.A., Doctoral student in Counseling Psychology, School of Education, Boston University

Andrea B. Goldschmidt, Ph.D., Assistant Professor, Department of Psychiatry and Behavioral Neuroscience, The University of Chicago

Amie E. Grills, Associate Professor in Counseling Psychology in the School of Education at Boston University

Lindsay S. Ham, Ph.D., Associate Professor and Director of Clinical Training, Department of Psychological Science, University of Arkansas, Fayetteville, AR

Keith C. Herman, Ph.D., Professor, Department of Educational, School, and Counseling Psychology, University of Missouri

Gillian Hewitt-Stubbs, Master's student in Clinical Psychology, School of Applied Psychology, Griffith University

Melissa K. Holt, Assistant Professor in Counseling Psychology in the School of Education at Boston University

Kimberly A.S. Howard, Ph.D., Associate Professor, Counseling Psychology, School of Education, Boston University

Kamilah B. Legette, M.A., Doctoral student in Human Development and Family Studies, University of North Carolina Greensboro

Daniel Le Grange, Ph.D., Professor, Department of Psychiatry, University of California, San Francisco

John E. Lochman, Ph.D., Professor, Clinical Psychology, The University of Alabama

Shawna Mastro, B.Psych., Clinical Psychology doctoral student, School of Applied Psychology, Griffith University

Paul C. McCabe, Ph.D., Professor, School Counseling, Counseling and Leadership, Brooklyn College of the City University of New York

Alexander J. Melkonian, Doctoral student in Clinical Psychology, Department of Psychological Science, University of Arkansas, Fayetteville, AR

Stuart B. Murray, Ph.D., Post-doctoral Fellow, Department of Psychiatry, University of California, San Diego

Thomas H. Ollendick, Ph.D., University Distinguished Professor, Department of Psychology, Virginia Polytechnic Institute

Lucia F. O'Sullivan, Ph.D., Professor, Department of Psychology, University of New Brunswick

V. Paul Poteat, Ph.D., Associate Professor, Department of Counseling, Developmental, and Educational Psychology, Lynch School of Education, Boston College

Nicole P. Powell, Ph.D., MPH, Research Psychologist, The University of Alabama Center for the Prevention of Youth Behavior Problems

Wendy M. Reinke, Ph.D., Associate Professor, Department of Educational, School, and Counseling Psychology, University of Missouri

Ian Rivers, Ph.D., Professor of Human Development, Department of Education, College of Business, Arts, and Social Sciences, Brunel University

Katelyn Rose, M.S.Ed., Master's student in School Psychology, Brooklyn College of the City University of New York

Zachary Rossetti, Ph.D., Assistant Professor in Special Education, School of Education, Boston University

Meghann K. Sallee, M.S., Doctoral student in Child Clinical Psychology, The University of Alabama

Janay B. Sander, Ph.D., Associate Professor, Department of Educational Psychology, Teachers College, Ball State University

Jillian R. Scheer, M.A., Doctoral student in Counseling Psychology, Department of Counseling, Developmental, and Educational Psychology, Lynch School of Education, Boston College

Elizabeth Swanson, Ph.D., Senior Research Associate, Meadows Center for Preventing Educational Risk, University of Texas at Austin

Andra Teten Tharp, Ph.D., Senior Health Scientist, Division of Violence Prevention, Centers for Disease Control and Prevention

Aaron M. Thompson, Ph.D., Assistant Professor, School of Social Work, University of Missouri

Sharon Vaughn, Ph.D., H.E. Hartfelder/Southland Corporation Regents Chair in Human Development, University of Texas at Austin

Melanie J. Zimmer-Gembeck, Ph.D., Professor, School of Applied Psychology, Griffith University and Menzies Health Institute of Queensland, Australia

INDEX

CPSIA information can be obtained
at www.ICGtesting.com
Printed in the USA
FFHW010719101118
49329096-53603FF